I0758609

Gianluca Tognon

50 POUNDS SLIMMER

Lose weight easily, without hoaxes

SUMMARY

FOREWORD

Have you always dreamed of losing weight quickly and easily? Have you tried a thousand diets or miraculous methods to lose the famous "seven kilos in seven days?" Where does the truth begin, and the hoaxes end?

My name is Gianluca Tognon. In this book, I will tell you how I've helped hundreds of men and women lose weight in a natural and balanced way, by helping them change their diet in a way that significantly improves both their health and mood.

I do not promise miracles, and I don't own a magic wand. Everything I've written in this book is based on scientific evidence, and my professional experience with hundreds of clients that I've worked with during the past fifteen years.

I won't offer you supplements or quick fixes and neither will I teach you a mantra that will make you lose weight if you promise to repeat it religiously. In this book you will find all the tips that have helped made my clients become fully independent in managing their diet.

With commitment and passion, you will also achieve excellent results, or even lose fifty pounds!

Gianluca Tognon

www.gianlucatognon.com

INTRODUCTION

It is a usual morning in Gothenburg, the Swedish city where I have lived for ten years. Outside my office window at Gothenburg University, I can see a gray sky that is common during winter- time. This year is quite unusual; it hasn't snowed yet.

The phone rings; it is a call from Lausanne.

A woman, head of human resources in a large food multinational company, is calling because she has some good news for me: after ten interviews, a trip to Lausanne to present my work and my ideas, a series of attitudinal tests, they had decided to offer me a job as a nutritional epidemiologist. They wanted to work with me and offered a salary of 6000 Swiss Francs a month. Among all the other candidates who had applied to this post, they had chosen me.

I could not believe this was happening to me.

After spending fifteen years as a researcher in Italy and seven years in Sweden, I'd finally landed the job of my dreams.

But this offer had a fundamental catch: I was supposed to sign an exclusive contract which would have allowed me to work only for their company. This meant closing down my blog, my YouTube channel and, most of all, no more dietary coaching with my clients. These conditions were non-negotiable. It was either take it or leave it.

This was not an easy call. I lost sleep for a couple of days, I talked to colleagues and friends. I thought extensively about this proposal, until eventually, I made my final decision: thank you very much for the proposal, it's a great honor, but I must refuse.

I could not throw the work I had done for many years under the bus, especially the brand I had built around my dietary coaching service, which was trusted by many people.After a few years, here I am. Writing this book about my experience.

Let me introduce myself. My name is Gianluca Tognon, I have been working in the nutritional field for many years, and I have books and scientific publications to my credit. Over the past ten years, I have helped hundreds of men and women regain control of their body weight and improve their health through a healthier diet.

I don't like trendy diets and, therefore, I do not advocate them. I respect the opinion of those who think the paleo, vegan, low-carb diets, or any other popular regime is the healthiest on earth. I don't believe you need to exclude food groups to eat healthily. I am instead convinced you need to include nutritious food into your meals. Popular diets are heavily promoted on social media and often gain a lot of followers. Many of the latter do not realize that most of these diets are usually based on two simple pieces of advice: cut added sugar and increase your vegetable intake. The exclusions they propose are just gimmicks that they usually justify by cherry picking scientific studies that support their hypothesis, while ignoring those studies that do not.I base my dietary advice on the principles of the Mediterranean diet, which (beware) has nothing to do with the commercial Italian diet which is full of foods rich in sugar and refined carbs. I described the results of my research studies on the Mediterranean diet's effects in a doctoral thesis that I defended at Westminster University in London.

This research project enabled me to publish several scientific publications, and even got me an invitation to speak at Harvard University in Boston, at Barilla in Italy. This made me gain several citations in the international press, including some in the Washington Post, the US Huffington Post, and The Telegraph.

A wealth of scientific data demonstrates the positive effects of the Mediterranean diet on human health. I am a strong advocate of the idea that, to prevent diseases with a healthy diet, you do not need to exclude certain foods or food groups. Instead, you need to upgrade your whole diet and eating style.The main merit of the eating style is that it is an easy one to follow! You do not need to make sacrifices. You can eat a variety of different foods and use them to prepare delicious dishes. I'll explain more about healthy cooking in the second section of this book.

At this point, you probably have a question in mind: can I really lose fifty pounds by following your advice? Well, yes. But be aware that losing weight is not only a matter of following a proper diet. It is above all, a matter of having the right mindset.

THE BASIC CONCEPTS TO EAT (AND THINK) BETTER

Why you are not losing weight

"Mr. B had been my client for a long time. He was a big man who walked with difficulty; his right meniscus was giving way under his weight, the tendons of the other leg had reached the limit, and it was a miracle that they had not yet torn apart. Mr. B had asked me for help to lose weight and improve his health. I checked the results of his most recent blood tests and created a personalized meal plan for him, encouraging him to do some physical exercise as well. I recommended a varied diet: fish, fruit, vegetables, and just a little red meat. I did not exclude any food as usual; I just recalibrated his portions.After a few months, he was even more overweight than before we had started working together. It was hard for him to understand why this was happening, and B had even more difficulty walking. My recommendations weren't working, but for what reason?

B swore that he had scrupulously followed every piece of advice I had given him and had been walking as much as possible.

Could his problems be more serious? A thyroid malfunction, perhaps?

I was doing everything I could for that patient; it was a professional blemish to have an overweight client who was gaining weight instead of losing it!

What did I do wrong? I kept asking myself.

After several months, I'd realized that it was useless (and even counterproductive) to insist; I had to live with the fact that I couldn't help him, and I eventually gave up. However, at the back of my mind, I couldn't help but think about this situation from time to time.Time erases everything, and I began to forget about Mr. B.'s case, but I still worked with another member of his family.

B was not the only one with a weight issue, his sister was also overweight, but my advice had worked perfectly in her case. And it was her who, many months later, finally told me, during a follow-up visit, what had happened to her brother.

"Mrs. B, the results we have obtained are excellent; I'm really sorry it didn't work the same way for your brother."

"Gianluca, it was not your fault. Nobody could help my brother. He is his worst enemy; he lied to everyone, even to himself. He said he was on a diet, but in reality, he increased his portions of food, had several snacks during the day, and ignored the advice you had given him. Recently, he had severe health problems and was hospitalized. Now he is on controlled feeding; he'll lose weight for sure."Here was the answer to the mystery of Mr. B, although I'm sorry that he ended up in the hospital.

Like many other people in your situation, after several attempts to lose weight, you have probably concluded that you can't succeed.

However, this is not necessarily true; you probably just took the wrong approach.

I have worked with many people who've wanted to lose weight for different reasons but could not obtain any results, or they could not maintain them. These people often followed the slimming diet of the moment, drank weight loss smoothies or took pills.

Slimming diets, drinks, or pills all come with one big drawback: they don't nourish your body.I lost count of the many people who told me, "I don't understand; I'm doing everything I know helps to lose weight, but my weight is the same, if not even higher!"

Several factors can explain why you can't lose weight. The most obvious one is that you don't exercise enough and that you eat more than necessary, as in Mr. B's case.

From a theoretical point of view, you will lose weight if the amount of calories burned is greater than the amount of calories ingested. Surprisingly though, I know many people who, after cutting their calorie intake and trained more often, still could not lose weight. However, I must add that, in my fifteen years of experience with dietary coaching, I have met very few people who could not lose weight after cutting their intakes and exercising even slightly more. My hypothesis is that most people have difficulties estimating how much food they're eating every day and end up eating more than they should while convincing themselves that they eat like a bird. It is not unusual that many of my clients come back to the first follow up visit and tell me they have been eating more than before and lost weight at the same time.In chapter X "Three steps to lose weight," I explain how you can reduce your daily food intake without feeling hungry. I will tell you how to prevent dehydration by drinking more water.

It is not always easy to estimate how much food you eat every day. A stressful life can lead to uncontrolled eating or increase your body fat stores as a consequence of an increased endogenous cortisol production. The latter hormone alters your metabolism and makes you accumulate fat mass. Many people live a stressful life today. A troubled job, a disabled parent, or a problematic relationship can make it difficult to find time to relax. How can you find more time for yourself? For starters, you need to accept that you will not be able to do everything and identify the tasks you can avoid, those you can do only occasionally, and the ones that you can delegate to other people. The table below will help you plan your tasks smartly.

Daily tasks (all)	Which ones can you skip or perform less frequently?	Which ones can you delegate?
Tasks connected to your job		
Home activities		
Family duties		
Other tasks		

Once you have identified the activities that you can occasionally do and the ones you can delegate to other people, you will have less tasks to do and more time for yourself. Which means you can dedicate your time to more anti-stress activities such as:

- Play with your children
- Walk in the park
- Listen to relaxing music while drinking herbal tea
- Go to a sauna or get a relaxing massage
- Take a nap
- Spend time with friends or family
- Call a friendDedicate yourself to your passions and many other activities!

When you are less stressed you usually eat more mindfully, and your body produces less cortisol. However, to fill in the table above is not the only thing you need to do; convince yourself that minimizing the amount of stress in your life is the best way to take care of yourself.

Some people feel guilty if they delegate what they perceive being their own responsibilities or errands to other people, but they do not realize that doing this will make more time for having deeper relationships with colleagues, partners, friends, and family members and, most of all, for themselves. You have no reason to feel guilty if you take the time to live a better life.

Lack of sleep is another crucial factor to consider in this discussion.

Negative thoughts and fears lead people to suffer from (usually temporary) insomnia, which generally ends when these problems get solved. If your sleep issues have been going on for a long time, you probably need professional help.

If your sleep quality is not optimal, these are some strategies that you can adopt:

Always go to sleep at the same time every night.

Follow a daily routine: e.g. take a bath, have an herbal tea, go to sleep.

Change the position in which you sleep.

Avoid mental taxing work before going to bed.

Turn on blue light instead of white light on your smartphone when you use it after 8 pm.

Avoid training during the last three hours before going to sleep.

Create a relaxing atmosphere in your bedroom: buy a comfortable mattress, sleep in a dark and quiet environment at a mild temperature.

Try aromatherapy by spraying a solution of essential oils on your pillow. Here is a recipe: mix ten drops of lavender, ten of clary sage, ten, twenty or thirty drops of chamomile, and fifteen of bergamot oil. You can also pour the essential oil mix into a cotton ball and place it on the nightstand.

- Use Bach flowers.
- If the noise bothers you, use earplugs.
- If you cannot switch all the lights, wear an eye mask.

Another factor that hinders weight loss is that your body accumulates visceral instead of subcutaneous body fat. Visceral fat tends to be more difficult to lose.Although in this book I focus more on losing weight without physical activity, I need to point out that, if you want to lose a significant amount of visceral fat, you usually need to implement an intense training program including three to four sessions every week.

Perhaps surprising to you, but another reason why you cannot lose weight is because you have too many distractions while eating. Eating while watching television or your smartphone will not allow you to concentrate on what you are putting into your stomach. Studies have shown a link between these behaviors and a greater likelihood of gaining weight. Turn off the TV and move your smartphone away when you are at the table and concentrate on what you are doing instead. Eat slowly and in a quiet environment. If you are not alone, talk to the people sitting at your table instead of watching television.

Another reason you don't lose weight is that you skip a meal even if you are hungry. If you do so and you end up starving, you will probably eat the food you have on hand, which is usually high in sugar and fat.

I don't think it's crucial to eat five meals a day. Three can be more than enough, two main meals and a smaller one. The two main meals could be breakfast and dinner, with a small lunch. In this case, the breakfast should be based on high-protein foods (eggs, cheese, yogurt) that help maintain satiety for a longer time. The key is to find the combination to stay full for a longer period of time, while eating less food. Alternatively, you could choose to eat a light dinner since during the night your body will not burn much energy while sleeping.

Another likely cause of your inability to lose weight is using medications that have side effects on your weight, such as antidepressants, antipsychotics, or medicines for bipolar disorder.

I obviously do not recommend interrupting your therapy, of course, but maybe you can talk to your doctor to see if you can take smaller doses. You can try to balance the drug's side effects by exercising more. Walk every day, hit the gym or the swimming pool more often. Counterbalancing the impact of the drug is essential because these drugs usually have substantial effects on body weight.

The last reason you can't lose weight, is because you are deficient in specific nutrients. As surprising as it might seem, you can have nutritional deficiencies even if you live in a country where the food is abundant! I always encourage new clients to do a blood test and check their nutrient levels. I usually notice a lack of vitamin D and iron that improves with a more nutritious diet and specific supplements.

THE PROBLEM OF
WEIGHT-LOSS DIETS

I'm sure everyone has some friends who have read a lot about how to lose weight and who have tried many diets promoted on the web or in the gym, thinking they will get great results. I know some people who prefer to spend an entire summer eating only chicken breast and white rice, thinking this will help them increase their muscle mass like the buffest guy at the gym. Once a week it's cheat time and they eat literally whatever they can find. I am horrified by these extreme behaviors, but those who choose them probably think that if you eat whatever you want once a week the body will not absorb it. Or similar nonsense. The source of this theory is generally the internet, where many diet gurus share their ideas on diet and nutrition, often with a huge conflict of interest because they also sell a lot of products. I am not sure everyone really understands the importance of getting reliable health information from an independent source or from someone who is only selling you his/her advice and not slimming products or supplements.

My point is that many popular diets are unhealthy and listening to improvising nutritionists' advice can have many negative consequences for your health.

Unfortunately, a lot of companies recruit thousands of salespeople to sell their slimming pills and supplements. Most of their salespeople do not have the education needed to give nutritional advice, and they just try to sell as many products as possible. On the web, you can also find stories of many people who were recruited as salespeople through pyramid schemes and who ended up broke after buying large stocks of supplements that they were never able to sell. I feel a lot of anger when I talk about these things because:

I cannot stand those who deceive people and exploit their need to find a job to make money. These pyramid marketing systems are a full-blown scam. Never agree to work with these companies. Many questionable methods are promoted as effective weight loss remedies when instead they only induce a temporary loss of body weight. Popular dietary programs ignore the specific needs that each individual person has. Many people think that anyone can be a nutritionist ignoring how improvising nutritionists contribute to spreading hoaxes. In this chapter, I want to talk about the problem of slimming diets, which are often prescribed by people who don't have the qualifications to do it. I have been working in the nutrition field for many years, and I have met hundreds of people who were utterly suffering from hunger! I'm talking about real hunger, not the emotional hunger that I will cover in chapter 5.

We know well how it works with many popular diets. You've probably tried them in the past: their main disadvantage is to drastically reduce your calorie intake for a while, subjecting you to long periods of restriction and... hunger! Many diets are also very monotonous, requiring you to eat a very limited number of foods until, eventually, you stop eating out of boredom. But can you continue like this? And for how long?

In this chapter, I would like to tell you more about these trendy diets that are commonly promoted by successful books that explain how to lose weight quickly and get back in shape without effort. These diets usually do not bring stable long-term benefits because all the lost weight will eventually come back. Some of them can even harm your health. The main reason these diets do not work is that they do not teach you how to eat correctly, for instance, they do not explain you which are the correct portions or how often you should eat different foods: how many times a week should you eat fish? And what about meat?

Trendy diets usually completely neglect these details. They do not provide nutritional education, but instead, they are hyper-simplified. It is also possible to consume large quantities of certain foods, usually protein and vegetables, without teaching you to feed yourself according to healthy nutrition rules. Very often, self-taught nutritionists who propose these diet plans pretend their remedies are based on the most recent scientific discoveries or that they have developed a working method after years of study and experience. In most cases, a quick look at the proposed meal plan reveals that it is just another low-carb diet. The latter is a diet developed in the 1960s (you got it, over sixty years ago!) by Dr. Atkins in the United States. Credit goes to Dr. Atkins for being the first to understand that carbohydrates (and not necessarily fat) played an essential role in weight gain. I also believe that a moderate reduction in carbohydrate intake can be helpful. Still, I also think that more than half a century after Atkins' discoveries, there are better ways to lose weight than completely exclude all carbohydrates. Not all carbohydrates and not all fats are necessarily the same and with the same physiological functions. In this book, I explain how the key is to replace "bad" carbohydrates with "good" fats.

Another critical factor of trendy diets is that, in many cases, these diets mostly consist of shakes and supplements. Once you stop using these products, you also stop losing weight and quickly regain the weight you have lost. Some diets promote the idea that specific food associations would allow a more rapid weight loss. Nothing could be more wrong than that! The only combination that makes sense from a nutritional standpoint is the combination of grains and legumes into the same meal (rice and lentils, millet and beans, etc.). This combination allows you to take a complete set of amino acids. The latter are the fundamental constituents of proteins. But apart from these two simple rules, I don't think there is much more from a scientific point of view, that justifies a particular attention to food associations.

Trendy diets are often unsustainable over time and are often also very expensive because they force you to buy specific products. The suggestions they provide are so extreme that it is impossible to continue for a long time, especially those that are high-protein diets very rich in meat and other protein foods. Other diets, however, restrict the number of calories drastically and make it impossible to adhere to them for a long time.

Trendy diets only aim to make money from the largest number of people as possible. Those who designed them are not interested in understanding your personal needs and they do not consider your potential health problems or your difficulty to digest large amounts of fiber. Not being able to consider your peculiarities, they are therefore not very useful. They do not consider your habits, your tastes, but they are hyper-simplified so that they can be adapted (read: sold) to everyone, even if they do not necessarily adapt to your specific case.

What to do then?

I believe that it is crucial to approach your weight problem from a completely different point of view. I explain to all my new clients how to reduce the sense of hunger, for example, by having a filling breakfast or by starting each meal with a "smart" salad. Although hunger is a physiological mechanism, it is possible to keep it under control. In the chapter "Three steps to lose weight" you will discover some tricks to make your meals more effective in stimulating a sense of fullness.

In general, meals that contain a lot of rapidly absorbed carbohydrates induce an increased secretion of insulin, resulting in a sudden drop in blood sugar after a short while. This mechanism leads to a rapid return of the sense of hunger. Instead of choosing foods that contain rapidly-absorbed carbohydrate (like white bread, desserts, etc.), you should aim to modulate your carbohydrate intake by choosing foods such as legumes that are not only a source of starch, but that are also rich in fiber, which slows down the absorption of carbohydrates and make hunger come back later. I think everyone who is trying to lose weight should focus on dealing with hunger. Curiously, many diets do not consider this factor, but they are rather exclusively focused on reducing fat, calories, or carbohydrates.

I think everyone should follow the official nutritional recommendations, which represent general guidelines valid for everyone, readapting this advice to suit your tastes and habits. A few evergreen rules that are always valid are: try to consume fruit and vegetables every day (five portions a day), reduce consumption of red and processed meat, and increase vegetable protein such as those derived from legumes and whole grains. Also, you should regularly consider nuts, fish, avocados (which are rich in healthy fats) and replace meat with products rich in vegetable protein. By reading this book, you will discover how to adopt these guidelines more effectively and cleverly.A fundamental aspect of healthy eating is to follow a specific order during each meal. You need to start with the least caloric and more satiating foods, up to the most caloric and less satiating ones, for example, you will be able to reduce the number of calories ingested without effort. This is a topic that we will cover in the chapter dedicated to the three steps to lose weight.

As the old saying goes, you should not throw the baby out with the bathwater. I must confess that my curious nature has led me to try to better understand the potential positive aspects related to trendy diets. It might seem to contradict what I have written so far in some cases it is still possible to get some good ideas even from popular diets. I have already mentioned Dr. Atkins and his discovery that carbohydrates play an essential role in regulating body weight. An evolution of his work was made by Dr. Barry Sears who, more recently, launched the Zone Diet. The concept is to consume macronutrients (carbohydrates, fats, and proteins) in "packages," more precisely defined as "zones " which swap carbohydrates for protein (40% carbohydrates, 30% protein and 30% fats, in terms of percentage of calories ingested). The zone diet made me think that it is possible to reduce the amount of carbohydrates without completely excluding them. If you have a sedentary lifestyle, a maximum of 40% of the calories you ingest should come from carbohydrates. This is an excellent compromise to reduce carbohydrates without banning them altogether. However, I can't entirely agree with Dr. Sears about raising the protein quota of the calories eaten. Instead, I think that approximately 40% of the calories consumed every day should come from healthy fats (such as those from fish and olive oil). This is the percent of fat that, in the traditional diet consumed in Crete (where the Mediterranean diet was born) contained. Anyway, I don't want to confuse you with all these calculations, especially because you won't have to do any of them. In this book I will explain how to reorganize you diet so that it will follow the rules above without making calculations.

Another popular myth is that, to lose weight, you need therapeutic and detoxifying fasts. In reality though, there are no ways to detoxify your body in a short time, just by fasting. When you do not eat for prolonged periods of time, your body begins to consume its muscle protein after a certain period. The result is that your bloodstream, especially your kidneys, will be "engulfed" by the nitrogen contained in all amino acids (i.e., protein building elements). Recently, Michael Mosley has devised a diet based on the so-called "alternating semi-fasting." His idea is that, to avoid the disadvantages of prolonged fasting, is to adopt a semi-fasting (500 calories per day for women and 600 calories per day for men) for one or two non-consecutive days every week (hence the name 5 + 2). According to Mosley, during the remaining days you can simply follow some generic rules for a healthy diet. For instance, eat fruits and vegetables and avoid overdoing it with refined cereals. Michael Mosley even goes so far as to argue that there are no rules for non-semi-fasting days. I think we can do better while limiting ourselves to 5-600 calories a day can be quite difficult for most people, the idea is not completely crazy. Generally, on Sundays, you sleep a little more. Why not take advantage of it to turn this day into a weekly detox by drinking mainly herbal teas, smoothies, or vegetable purees and excluding the most caloric foods such as refined cereals and sweets? It can't harm for sure, and there is no risk of burning muscle protein, given that we are talking about one day (maximum two) a week.

THE HIDDEN ENEMY THAT MAKES YOU GAIN WEIGHT

I remember one day when I was sitting in my office with Mrs. M, a new client. M was a business- woman who had a company that provides aid to motorists whose car stops working in the middle of a journey by sending mechanics and tow trucks. Her job was 24-7 and M often had to remain in her office until late at night to supervise the work of her employees, especially on weekends.

It was evident that this work rhythm was damaging Mrs. M. With these rhythms, you would expect someone to lose weight, while M continued to gain weight. My task was to understand why. She slept only three to four hours per night, and commonly drank a lot of coffee. When my patient mentioned how much coffee she was drinking every day, a light bulb went on in my head. I had to investigate this issue.

"Mrs. M, on average, how many coffees do you drink every day?"

"Lots, at least twenty. I sleep only a few hours, and I'm stressed. I can't work without coffee."

“It's not a good thing; that's far too many. Do you add sugar into your coffee? "

“Yes. I put one teaspoon of sugar in each cup of coffee."

I had found the key to the problem. Here's what made Mrs. M gain: sugar!

Is a single teaspoon of sugar that bad? Not necessarily, but let's do the math.

One teaspoon of coffee is about ten grams of sugar.

Twenty cups of coffee means twenty teaspoons of sugar, more than a pound of sugar a day, and only to sweeten your coffee!

Each gram of sugar contains 4 kcal, 400 kcal per day, and about 12 000 kcal per month, just because you don't like your coffee bitter!

Mrs. M was genuinely shocked by that revelation. Unknowingly she was taking in a disproportionate amount of sugar, and what's worse was that she didn't think this was a problem.

This story has a moral: often the enemy (who makes us gain weight) does not appear to us only in the form of junk food or very large portions, but also in small things. "The devil is in the detail." Well, that's true for fattening food.

Of course, I immediately told Mrs. M to cut out both coffee and sugar, and she obtained the results she wanted.

Do you feel like you have an enemy whose name you don't know, but who continually tries to sabotage all your attempts to lose weight? Well, this enemy is not imaginary; it exists! It's sugar. Probably, like many other people I've helped lose weight over the past fifteen years, you're thinking, *but I don't use a lot of sugar!*

Maybe not. Or maybe so.

Start counting the number of spoons of sugar you use every day (or the number of sweet treats): four of five per day? To eat as little as 50 g of sugar per day (i.e., the equivalent of five tablepoons of sugar) might seem little. However, fifty grams of sugar correspond to 4600 calories per month! Now maybe you are starting to see the danger of using too much sugar in a different light.

But that is not all. The sugar you put into your coffee is not the only one that you should worry about. Sucrose is a ubiquitous additive used in many foods, even those advertised as healthy. Breakfast cereals contain added sugar, many yogurts are sweetened, especially the low-fat and non-fat ones, which, are not necessarily no-sugar as well, unfortunately. Even some pasta sauces are sweetened, as is balsamic vinegar. Incredible, isn't it?

To realize the extent of this mass poisoning of which we are all victims of, try to do the experiment I recommend to all new clients: go to the supermarket and check the labels of what you're thinking to buy. How many products, even unsuspected ones, contain sugar? The correct answer is too many!

Sugar does not induce satiety; it makes you eat more and serves the only purpose to treat your palate. Eliminate it from your diet, even trying to always check labels by buying products that do not contain it. You probably remember what I'd mentioned in the previous chapter, i.e. that the main benefit associated with my weight loss programs is to learn how to control your hunger and increase satiety. Sugar does not give you satiety. On the contrary, it makes you eat more, and this is precisely the goal that the food industry aims for: making you consume (and therefore buy) a greater quantity of their products.

Sugar is just one of many hidden enemies that can destroy all your weight loss efforts. In most cases, each of us does not eat because of hunger, real or nervous as it is. We eat out of habit, because we are in the company of someone (friends, relatives, etc.), because we are bored, or because we are attracted by a specific product with captivating packaging. When you eat while being distracted, you don't realize what is going down into your stomach. Each of us every day makes an average of two hundred fifty decisions regarding food. Should I eat oranges or apples? Meat or fish? Think about it. There are so many occasions when you think about food, even if you are not aware of it.

It is not easy to be completely aware of how much food you eat every day. Therefore, I would like to teach you five easy rules that will help you eat in a more mindful way and regulate the "flow" of calories into your stomach. Here they are:

1. Define your danger areas: identify those situations that make you lose control of what you eat and try to avoid them.
2. Replace 20% of what you eat wisely.
3. Leave the pot in the kitchen and serve the already portioned dishes on the table.
4. Don't deprive yourself of comfort food completely.
5. Be wary of foods promoted as healthful.

Are you still confused? Let's analyze these five tips a little more in detail.

Define your danger areas

What are your "danger areas?" In what situations do you find yourself most likely to eat without controlling what you are doing? Here are four common examples:

- When you shop your food.
- When you think of having a snack.
- When you eat out.
- When you eat at your desk.

In the case of the "shopping" danger area, I would like to give you three pieces of advice. The first, most obvious one, is never shop for food when you are hungry. By doing this, you risk buying more food than you need. The second tip is to bring a shopping list with you every time you go to a food shop or supermarket. Your list should include only the foods you need. In the second part of this book, I will also tell you how to make a smart shopping list. The third and final piece of advice to redefine your danger areas is to stop buying foods that are harmful to your health or limit the amount you purchase by a lot. I'm talking about sweet products, carbonated drinks, salty snacks, or processed meat such as cured meats, canned meat, etc. These foods, once they enter your pantry, will have preferential access to your stomach. Try to avoid buying them altogether.

The decision to snack is another potential risk area. When you are hungry, and you have a few choices, you risk eating high-calorie junk, usually because those few options that are available are sweet or salty snacks. How can you redefine this risk area? Regularly purchase a certain amount of fruit, nuts, natural yogurt without sugar, and maybe some whole meal biscuits. Lupins (unsalted) are also a possibility. Keep these foods handy at home or in the office, so you don't have a problem with a healthy snack.

A vital area of danger to your diet is undoubtedly all meals you have outside your home. It is not always easy to control what you eat when you are in a restaurant, or when you dine at someone else's house. Here is a practical list of tips that will help you keep the meals you consume away from home under control:

- Avoid, as far as possible, buffets and "all you can eat" restaurants, where you can, in theory, eat until you drop.   Start each meal with a salad.
- Eat at the same pace of the person who is eating the slowest among those who are sitting at your table excluding children (who are often very slow). Avoid pre-ordering the whole

meal at the beginning when you are hungry. Instead, start by ordering a dish (after a salad) and, if you are still hungry, consider sharing a portion of another dish with another person.   Try to avoid, or at least limit, the amount of bread, breadsticks, and other sources of refined carbohydrates you eat (such as pasta, potatoes, gnocchi, etc.).   If possible, start your meal with a broth: it will fill up your stomach and make you eat less of other dishes.   Give preference to fish and order the one cooked with less fat (grilled, baked in foil, etc.).   Ask questions about cooking methods: if they use a lot of oil, if the ingredients are breaded, etc. Try to understand which courses are less caloric than the others.

Another danger area is the office. Apart from the discussion above about snacks to keep at hand, make sure you have access to a water bottle, which you can keep on your desk. To always have water at your hands allows you to keep your body hydrated and, to some extent, your belly full. Try to bring home-cooked meals from home as much as possible and keep a bottle of olive oil to dress your salad.

Replace 20% of what you eat intelligently

We all tend to underestimate our portion sizes. Whenever you are about to put food on your plate, estimate your portion size, then reduce it by about 20% (one fifth) and replace this amount with lower-calorie ingredients like vegetables, legumes, or fruit. For example, instead of preparing 100 g of pasta and oil, prepare 80 g with 20 g of vegetables. If you want, you could do even better (50-50), but you may feel like you are eating too little. By following the 20% rule, however, you will hardly realize that you are eating less, and you will have saved, in the case of pasta, 70 kcal.

Leave the pot in the kitchen and serve the dishes with the food already dosed on the table

A widespread habit in my home country is to bring the pot to the table so that the diners can help themselves. Well, that's another way we overeat without noticing. It's best to pre-portion the food on each plate before bringing it to the table, so you're sure to eat the correct amount. Finally, place all leftovers in the refrigerator or freezer divided into individual portions to reduce the possibility of consuming excess food later.

Don't deprive yourself of comfort food completely

Many diets fail because they deprive you of the foods you like best. I am aware that I usually discourage sugar consumption. However, so-called "comfort" foods (usually sweets, but everyone has their own) are not necessarily 100% prohibited. The important thing is to have a rule and change your eating habits not to feel completely deprived of the foods you like most. Generally, my rule of thumb is to have a couple of desserts a week, choosing the least elaborate ones or those made at home without sugar. You can have a cheat meal of your choice once a week, which could be pizza or a large steak, whatever you like best. Once a month, you could add a further cheat meal, and eat something you like a lot but at the same time has too many calories to be consumed frequently. For example, my monthly tear is the McDonald's sandwich, which I eat strictly together with a sugar-free drink. As you can see, I have my weaknesses, too!

Finally, comfort foods aren't all necessarily bad. For example, I recently discovered a Swedish brand of oat milk (Oatly) that I like a lot and that I use when I want to indulge myself. The top is when I drink it after shaking it vigorously and its foams a lot. I also recently found that I love it even more mixed with soluble barley. Seeing is believing!

Be wary of foods promoted as healthy

Here's a very "slippery" risk area: the foods that look healthy but are nothing but healthy. I have already explained extensively how breakfast cereals and yogurt are both examples of potentially healthy food which are unfortunately often filled with added sugar by producers, which dilutes most of their health benefits. This problem is very common with low-fat foods where fat is removed (and, in the case of dairy products, sold as cream) and replaced with sugar (which is an inexpensive ingredient). Dairy cream is way more expensive than sugar; therefore, you can see why this is a good bargain for the food industry (but not for your health). Other foods at risk, because they are considered healthy, are highly processed organic foods that also contain lots of fat, salt, or added sugar. Salami and hams, canned organic fruit, and many other products are in some cases labeled as "organic" because their ingredients were not treated with either antibiotics or pesticides, but still belong to health risk categories. Avoid them or consume them occasionally. Finally, sugar-free drinks and desserts with added artificial sweeteners do not contain calories, they are not carcinogenic as many people think, but they can still be addictive because of their sweet taste. They could accustom the palate to a taste so "sugary" that you will want even more of it. Again, be very careful.

I think you have understood that hidden dangers are many, but after reading this chapter, I hope you have acquired the tools to avoid the traps and the many pitfalls that lurk in everyday life. In the next chapter, I will tell you how you are self-sabotaging your attempts to lose weight. Don't you think this is possible? Read, and you will find that, unfortunately, this is the case!

HOW YOU ARE SELF-SABOTAGING YOUR WEIGHT LOSS ATTEMPTS

L et me tell you a story that perfectly represents an unattainable goal. My favorite story is that of Icarus and his attempt to reach the sun.

Icarus and his father Daedalus, creator of the famous Labyrinth, had been imprisoned within it by King Minos, who did not want anyone to discover the Labyrinth's secrets. Daedalus devised a way to escape, combining feathers with wax, making wings. Thanks to this solution, he and his son Icaro were able to fly out of prison.

The son, as excited as he was by this experience, wanted to reach an even more ambitious goal: he wanted to reach the sun. But he did not consider that the heat of the sun's rays would quickly melt the feathers' wax. Icarus fell into the sea and died.

What can we learn from this story? The take-home message is that trying to reach an unattainable goal is always the wrong choice and can even sabotage your attempts to reach this goal. Icarus did not think about the effect of the sun's rays, he was only focused on reaching a very ambitious goal. In a way then, he has self-sabotaged himself, by underestimate the danger that eventually killed him.

Now think about your (several) attempts to lose weight. Why do you often fail? In many cases, you have probably tried to reach unattainable goals, and, instead of facing the fact that your goal was overambitious, you ended up self-sabotaging your attempt to lose weight. After a while, you probably started to notice that your self-control diminished, and you began to steer more and more away from the program you had set for yourself.

These are harmful behaviors, which you absolutely must avoid in order not to end up like Icarus. After all, nobody likes to fall treacherously to the ground, do they?

In this chapter, I would like to discuss a crucial topic that concerns a type of behavior I have observed in many people, namely the self-sabotage of your attempt to lose weight. It may seem incredible to you, but you can do this: on one hand, you have the will to live a healthier life and lose weight, but on the other hand, you unconsciously sabotage all your attempts, making your efforts pointless.

First, I would like to discuss a few situations that I have often observed while working with my clients and try to give you some useful advice to avoid making the same mistakes.

One reason why you are probably self-sabotaging yourself is because you are giving yourself unrealistic weight loss goals. Also, you are probably not considering an appropriate time frame. Many people who contact me for a health consultation tell me that they would like to lose forty, sixty, or even eighty pounds! I usually explain to them that they can achieve such an ambitious goal, but only in a prolonged time frame, during which the enthusiasm may even die out. What I recommend to these people (and also to you if you find yourself in this situation) is to set a more realistic goal. For example, 10% of your weight, and give yourself a realistic time interval, for example, five to six months. In a reasonable time, you will already be able to celebrate your first milestone, and this will give you more confidence in your ability to continue your weight loss journey.

The second reason you are most likely sabotaging your attempts to lose weight is because you might be eating too little. It is incredible how many people still think that, to lose weight, you almost have to fast. Well, not really! Many of my clients tell me that, after following the meal plan that I've assigned them, they tend to eat more than before. I must say that this does not surprise me. It does not surprise me because, for example, I recommend they increase the amount of fruits and vegetables they consume, and I suggest consuming more vegetable protein and not just animal protein. If you follow the advice in this book, you will soon realize that you are consuming fewer calories while eating more. Eating too little or semi-fasting does not help you; on the contrary, it hinders you because it makes your path scarcely sustainable over time. To set an overambitious goal can sabotage your attempt to lose weight, which will then inexorably fail.

A similar situation is when you avoid eating foods that could help you lose weight because you believe they make you fat. Examples of foods you might erroneously think will make you gain weight are high-fat foods such as nuts, which instead allow you to reduce the sense of hunger, and some protein foods, but which also contain starch, such as legumes. These foods are not only healthy, but they are precious allies of maintaining a healthy weight. Do not be afraid to consume them regularly as a snack or in a salad. Your weight will benefit, and you will feel the sense of satiety quicker and more easily. Extra virgin olive oil is also a calorie rich food, but it is extremely rich in antioxidants and substances beneficial for your health. If you want to indulge in it, reduce the portion of carbohydrate dishes instead. It is always better to eat less pasta but topped with more olive oil than the other way! Finally, bananas deserve a separate discussion. Among the various types of fruits to choose from, this is one of the most caloric. However, it also has an excellent satiating power. I recommend it as a snack before going to the gym because it helps maintain a more stable blood sugar level. I would avoid eating it just every day (unless I go to the gym every day), but I wouldn't exclude it from the healthy food list anyway.

The third reason you may probably be sabotaging yourself in some way is that you are not asking for help. Aside from the obvious advice to go to a professional for tips on how to eat healthily, there are other ways you can get help from other people. You can ask your family to support you, for instance, by asking them to help you cook or to shop for healthier groceries like fruit, nuts, fish, or vegetables. Getting help from family members allows you to make your life easier, but it is also a way to help them to eat better, too. It is vital to ask friends and family not to hinder you in your weight-loss path, explaining to them how important it is to you.

Another good idea is to partner with another person who also wants to lose weight. Besides going out for a walk together, you can agree on your goals together and celebrate when you reach them. You can also support each other when you can't achieve one of these goals. Mutual encouragement with another person with whom you share some common goals will be your best weapon. Together with this person, you will be able to keep what I call the "weight accounting," keeping track of the goals you have achieved.

In the context of your relationships with others, it is worth having a separate discussion with the people you surround yourself with. In this case, it is not a question of self-sabotage, but the fact of insisting on associating with "saboteurs" is not healthy anyway. There are generally two types of "saboteurs" who say, "Come on, are you really on a diet, AGAIN?" They will not stop bothering you until you swallow 3,000 calories in one evening (often under the form of alcohol), and if you don't do so, you are not one of them. Another type of "saboteurs" is represented by those who instead comment on every small change in your body weight, even if only 100 g. I know I'm dealing with an unpleasant subject, but the type of people we want to surround ourselves with is often up to us to decide. In the case of the "competition swallowers," I believe I don't need to clarify why you should try to see them a little less frequently. Now and then, a meal that is larger than usual or a bit more of alcohol than what you're used to can be good for the spirit, but the systematic gulping is instead dangerous. As for the second group of "saboteurs," in all sincerity, I struggle to understand how it is possible to consider these people friends who continually show appreciation or comments on your physical appearance. In general, these people serve only the purpose of increasing your obsession with your body. An obsession that, let's face it, you don't need! Be selective when you decide who you hang out with; there is no shortage of opportunities to meet new people, perhaps with ideas more similar to yours in terms of food. Have you ever checked out events on Meetup.com? It's a platform that many people use to meet new friends and enjoy fun activities together. Try it, and I am sure you will find some new friends who have neither an obsession with compulsive binging nor an obsession with your physical appearance. These people exist, trust me!

Another situation, also quite common, is self-sabotage. Don't allow negative thoughts and your mind stop you on your journey to losing weight. For example, you convince yourself that you will never succeed in your intent of losing weight, and you get depressed thinking that what you are doing to reach this goal is not enough. You tell yourself that you are not strong enough, that you do not have enough motivation. All these negative thoughts are going to sabotage all your attempts to lose weight. One mistake that should be avoided is comparing yourself to others. We are not all the same, and for some people losing weight may be easier than it is for you. It is not necessarily true that you will fail or are "inferior" to your friend who is slimmer than you. Your body, genetics, commitments, and problems are different, and so is your way of losing weight. Maybe you need more time, perhaps more effort, but don't let the comparison with others demoralize you. Compare yourself with your previous situation, a month or a year ago. Doing this allows you to evaluate successes and failures more objectively. Remember, never compare yourself to others. Instead, try to be pleased with your progress.

Speaking of negative thoughts, many people feel in the spotlight because of their physical appearance. I'm not a psychologist, but I think it's essential to learn not to worry too much about judgment from other people. Don't be afraid to let others down if you struggle to lose weight; it's your challenge, not theirs. If you are trying to lose weight to please others (because you feel you're under a spotlight), you will not easily reach your goal because the reason you have chosen is not personal enough. Stop doing this and try to understand why losing weight is important to you; think of a pleasant reason of why you want to lose weight, such as feeling less bulky when you walk around, reduce the sense of breathlessness you have every time you move, and live long enough to see your grandchildren graduate. Choose a personal and rewarding reason to make you want to lose weight and maintain it over time.

Before closing this chapter, I would like to mention some other everyday situations that might sabotage your attempts to lose weight. The first one is to not wear too much clothing during the wintertime. Some people are, by nature, a bit chilly but forget that a bit of cold wheather makes your body burn more energy. Obviously,

I'm not suggesting that you walk around in shorts in the middle of winter, but at least try not to over-cover your body. And don't be afraid to go out for a walk even if the temperature is below zero; if you walk at a steady pace, you will see that you will warm up quickly. Trust me, I live in Sweden!

The last form of self-sabotage I would like to mention is a little tricky. Over the years I have seen many people modify their diet because of what some "specialists" (or presumed such) had told them. Often these people base their dietary advice on genetic or molecular tests that have little or no scientific grounds. Some of these tests are supposed to identify food intolerances, despite there are no reliable methods to evaluate adverse reactions to food, except for gluten intolerance due to celiac disease or lactose intolerance. I have seen many people exclude many healthy foods because they were told they could not "tolerate" them. Don't be fooled by these scams!

Also, as incredible as it might be, there are still many people that in 2021 believe to the beneficial effects of saunas on weight loss or that you can lose weight by using slimming algae, supplements, slimming bands, and many others unconventional methods. If you are taking supplements or pills, unless prescribed by a specialist, they will not help you lose weight. To add insult to injury, taking pills will make you shift your attention away from the lifestyle changes you need because, in your mind, you will picture the pills doing all the work for you. As you can easily imagine, unfortunately, this cannot be the case. A commitment on your part is required even when these pills are prescribed by a dietologist (a physician specializing in dietetics). You are the real architect of your success. It is your challenge.

I hope I have given you some good food for thought and the tools you need to reach your ideal weight. Now you have a better understanding of why (perhaps unknowingly) you have always sabotaged all your attempts to lose weight with your behavior. It is essential to know yourself well before facing any new challenge.

RECOGNIZE AND DEFEAT EMOTIONAL HUNGER

"I have spoken several times about emotional hunger, and in this chapter, I want to go a bit deeper into this discussion. The first thing I want to tell you is to avoid underestimating it. Emotional hunger can ruin many people's health and weight loss attempts.

Psychologists are working to better understand this issue. Among the latter, I would like to recommend Susan Albers' books, one of the best-known professionals in this field. Dr. Albers' books inspired me while writing this chapter[1].

In this section, I will explain what you can do when you find yourself experiencing that strong desire to either eat whatever you can find or to eat a specific food, usually a sweet treat.

Let's start with some simple common-sense tips, the first of which is quite apparent: don't buy those foods you already know that will make you lose control: chocolate, sweets, etc.

It won't be easy to resist to them, you already know that; therefore, it's better to avoid buying them.Another essential tip is to look for distractions when hunger appears out of the blue. The latter is one of the characteristics of emotional hunger. Get out and go for a walk. To distract yourself helps you release stress, one of the known causes of emotional eating. Walk around a bit and get a breath of fresh air, and

---

[1] Susan Albers, 50 Ways to Soothe Yourself Without Food. New Harbinger Publications, Inc.

think about something fun, like which countries to visit on your next vacation!

Try to eat enough at meals. Many of my clients tell me they eat more after they've started following my dietary tips than before. If you consume your meals regularly and do not limit yourself excessively, you will avoid continually feeling hungry all day, which is usually a condition that will make you end up eating whatever food you have on hand. And the most available foods are usually sweet, salty snacks and so on.

But let's get to the heart of the discussion. It is essential to learn to distinguish emotional hunger from real hunger. Only the latest indicates that your body needs nourishment. Many of the people who have asked me for weight loss advice in the past, often told me, "I'm always hungry, I'm constantly hungry." One piece of advice I give all my clients is: Have you ever thought about analyzing your hunger? The answer is usually, "No, actually not. In what sense should I analyze my hunger?"

The first, real advantage of my method is that I invite everyone to stop for a moment to think and learn to recognize their body's signals. Stop, count to ten every time you get hungry, and see if the urge persists. Very often, a hunger attack hides other needs, for example, the need to distract yourself for a moment and relax, an anxiety attack, or the simple desire to break free from boredom, perhaps because you have been working or studying for several hours without a pause. Hunger is often a signal that your body is sending you because it wants you to take care of it, even if only for a minute or two.

How can you distinguish between emotional hunger and real hunger? First of all, wait ten seconds before you even consider eating some food. During this time, reflect on whether your hunger is real, and you will be surprised by how many times it is not. You might realize that you only ate an hour before. Get used to doing this exercise regularly before eating something.There are some guidelines to distinguish physiological hunger from emotional hunger. Real hunger comes slowly; it doesn't appear as if you switched an on/off button; the latter phenomenon is typically a sign of an emotional hunger attack. If you see your hunger ignite as the engines of a space rocket, what you are experiencing will probably be emotional hunger and not real hunger. Often the trigger that activates this sensation is a situation that makes you feel anxious, or worried. More simply, you have just watched your colleagues eat something that makes your mouth water.

Another feature that can help you identify physiological (real) hunger is to have a rumbling belly. Real hunger comes slowly, and at some point, you start to feel that your stomach is sending you some signs that its empty.

The following table will help you distinguish between the two types of hunger described above. Always remember to count to ten before deciding whether to eat or not, and in these ten seconds, "analyze" your hunger as shown below.

How to distinguish between:	
Emotional hunger	**Real, physiological hunger**
It arrives suddenly as if activated by an on/off button.	Gradually increases as meals are spaced out.
It arises quickly in response to external stimuli, for example, when someone announces that they want to buy ice cream.	You have symptoms that indicate a need for food, such as belly rumbling.
It increases in situations of psychophysical stress.	You spontaneously stop eating when you reach satiety.
You eat compulsively without even tasting food.	You can wait a while before you sit down at the table.
You crave a particular type of food, typically sweets, or chocolate.	You feel the need to eat something to fill your belly, not a specific food.
It is difficult to achieve a feeling of satisfaction after you have eaten.	The feeling of having a full stomach increases as you eat.
After eating you feel guilty.	You have no sense of guilt after eating.

But why do we eat? The most obvious answer is to nourish our body so that it doesn't have to feed on itself. In reality, this is not always the case. We all eat because of negative thoughts and emotions, making us eat more than we need or without being hungry. Unfortunately, positive feelings can also lead to overeating. Sometimes you eat because the food makes you feel good, and you don't want this feeling to stop.

Eating puts you in a sort of trance state. It makes you feel good and gives you a sense of relief. Eating is a way to relax and to kill boredom. Quoting the American psychologist Susan Albers who I've mentioned above, "Use the power of your mind to become aware of your need to eat in a new way. Embrace your food craving and get to know it. Investigate your need to eat uncritically." Let's analyze three strategies that will allow you to eat more consciously and give you comfort, even without food.

Strategy no. 1: Keep a diary

Writing down your problems (the so-called narrative therapy) is a simple and clinically proven way to help soothe your psyche. It helps to understand your feelings and to see them from a different perspective. Unexamined feelings and emotions can drag you in unwanted directions. Writing down your thoughts can help you reconsider your situation more realistically and positively. Above all, when you reread what you wrote after a few days, you may achieve mental serenity and realize that you were seeing things with more criticism than necessary.

Some advice for effective journal writing Plan to write at the same time every day and start by writing one or two notes a day.

Write without worrying about typos or grammar mistakes (free association) and for each entry in your diary, describe your emotions in the past (yesterday I felt), present (today I feel that) and future (tomorrow I would like to feel).

On the internet, you can find some websites which offer online diary tools.

Here are three steps that, if followed every day, will allow you to keep an effective and useful diary and to get the most out of narrative therapy.

Step n. 1: Start writing your emotions.

If you don't know how to do this, here are some ideas to get started:

- The worst thing about this situation is that ...
- Three adjectives that best describe how I feel right now are
- The reason I feel this emotion is ...
- When I eat, I feel ...

Step n. 2: Stimulate positive thinking

After finishing with the first step and writing down your past, present, and future feelings or thoughts, choose one of the following statements and start writing a few lines about:

- A joyous moment or a fun time you had in the past.
- A time when you felt at peace or experienced intense calmness.
- An occasion when you felt completely relaxed.
- A day when you had a strong spirit of adventure, for example, when you tried something new, like scuba diving.

Step n. 3: Add some wisdom to your thoughts

Take advantage of the positive mood you reached during the previous step and start reconsidering the thoughts and feelings you reported during the first step in a different way. Try to have a more realistic view of your life: Are you exaggerating your negative feelings? Think about how you can recreate positive emotions following these few steps more often.

Strategy no. 2: Take advantage of the other senses

You don't necessarily need to eat something to calm your mind. You can use the other four senses in many different ways. Let's see how.

Smell

Using aromatherapy is an excellent idea. Buy some herbs or incense and create a scented environment at home or while taking a bath. Buy pleasant scents and diffusers, especially in the bedroom. Try choosing a different aroma for every room.

View

Even your sight can give you pleasant sensations that help your mind to relax. Watch a fun video on YouTube or a video from your last vacation. Look at images like photos of friends and family, pictures of landscapes or of places you'd like to visit. Look at the paintings you have at home as if you were in a museum. If you don't have paintings, you can hang pictures.

Touch

Petting your pet or a soft toy is an action that gives you pleasant sensations that help you relax. Alternatively, you can take a hot bath or go to the sauna, after which you can practice self-massage. Online you can find some examples of how to do it. Finally, wrap yourself in a blanket or purchase an electric tool to warm your feet. A practical and useful idea is to buy a stress reliever doll to squeeze when you feel nervous.

Hearing

Listening to relaxing music is a great way to release the tension of a busy day. You can also listen to an audiobook or podcast to learn a new topic (e.g., a language). You can find several interesting podcasts on Spotify.

Buy an inexpensive indoor Zen fountain and use it to create a soothing sound. Finally, if you can, isolate yourself from the outside world for half an hour with earplugs.

Strategy no. 3: Find someone to share mutual comfort with

Choose a friend or a colleague who can listen and talk to you without judgements. Agree to call this person when, for instance, you feel that emotional hunger is coming. You can choose a code word to notify each other when you need help.

Invite this person to encourage you from time to time and spontaneously via email or voice message. Try to listen carefully to the other person and focus on everything you are being told. Meet regularly or at least call each other regularly. Set limits, it is okay to decline to talk when you can't be available.

Give each other feedback using the "sandwich" technique: start with a positive comment (e.g., it is good that you did not eat sugar yesterday), continue with the specific advice (e.g., if you want to continue like this, you can try to prepare a sugar-free dessert using this recipe), and conclude with an encouraging message (e.g., if you keep it up, you will soon be able to avoid sugar-rich foods). Reward yourself and celebrate your progress together. If no one you know is suitable to join you on this journey, you can also find a pen pal or join an online virtual support group.

More tips

Here are other ideas that will help distract you from the sense of hunger:

- Go shopping for inexpensive items.
- Volunteer for an NGO.
- Do some knitting or crochet, or another do-it-yourself.
- Laugh. Read, watch, listen, think of something funny.

The techniques indicated above represent your "toolbox," keep them at hand and use the best one that suits the various situations.

REVITALIZE YOUR METABOLISM

An active metabolism is essential to lose weight and stay healthy. The best way to boost your metabolism is to have an active lifestyle of more physical activity or to play sports. I still remember when I combined business with pleasure, doing sports, and eating Belgian chocolate without any remorse.

How did I do it?

Well, my life sometimes involves traveling between Sweden and Italy. It is a long and tiring journey, I often have to change planes, and it is at a time when I feel emotional hunger starting to manifest itself.

Luckily, I discovered a fantastic thing at Brussels airport: ecological chargers that are activated by pedaling! I swear, when I saw them for the first time I didn't believe it: I don't appreciate the exercise bike (I prefer to run in open spaces, it's much more fun), but I liked the idea, it was ecological and allowed me to do physical activity while keeping my metabolism active.

The charging of the phone while exercising has become my routine every time I fly through Brussels airport. Thanks to this trick, I can train, turn on my metabolism, and treat myself with some Belgian chocolates without any sense of guilt!

In this chapter, I will answer a question that is frequently asked of me, namely: "How can I revitalize my metabolism?" I imagine that many times you, too, have thought that your metabolism has actually stopped, or maybe you even believe that it has stopped forever. Well, that's not the case. There are ways to stimulate your metabolism and give it a push forward to burn more calories and thus promote weight loss.

Unfortunately, this is one of those cases in which it is difficult not to have to resort to physical activity and this is because, if you want to revitalize your metabolism, the best way to go is to increase your muscle mass.

It is your muscle mass that burns the energy from sugar, and fat you get from your diet. Burning more will allow your metabolism to increase its efficiency. The best thing to do to gain muscle mass is to join a gym, practice strength training, or do the same types of exercises, such as push-ups and lifting weights, at home.

If you don't have much time for physical activity, try an app called "7 Minute Workout," which will allow you to allocate seven minutes of strength training every day. The exercises are quite intense, and this will undoubtedly enable you to gain some muscle. Seven minutes is a very short time so, there's no excuse for not having any time, okay? You can start installing this app right away and start doing more exercise, or you can go to the gym a few times a week to gain even more lean mass.

Another way to stimulate your metabolism when it seems it has entirely fallen asleep, is to increase your protein intake. The latter will also have an indirect effect on muscle mass, especially if you start to train regularly. We Italians tend to consume many carbohydrates; we are very fond of pasta, pizza, and so on. However, to eat a lot of carbs, especially from refined sources, is not the best way to build muscle. Instead, proteins are essential because they help us burn more energy and are crucial muscle mass constituents. What are the sources of protein? First of all, legumes which you can add to recipes of pasta, rice, millet, or other cereals (e.g., couscous) or cereal-like such as buckwheat or quinoa. Replacing half of your usual portion of grains with the same amount of legumes allows you, on one hand, to consume less sugar and on the other hand, to increase your protein consumption.

Another important source of protein is dairy products, especially cheese. Unfortunately, the latter has often been demonized, despite being a food that is not only good but also very healthy. Studies (including the ones I've published with my colleagues in Sweden) show that it is not such an unhealthy food as many people believe. You can consume three small portions a week of cheese (50-80 g) without worrying about any negative health effects: Give preference to the aged ones which contain less lactose (or none at all) and allows you to take in a high amount of good quality protein and calcium, both of which are essential constituents of your bones.

As for meat, you don't need to eliminate it completely. Give preference to white meat at the expense of red and processed meat. The latter includes canned meat, cured meats, etc. As a rule of thumb, you can consume a couple of servings of white meat per week and one portion of red meat. As for processed meat, not more than once a month is ideal.

Another way to increase your protein intake is to use whey protein, which represent another useful tool for increasing lean mass. One scoop per day, roughly equivalent to 10 g of protein, dissolved in water or milk will help you increase your lean mass. Try to use whey protein during a period when you are exercising and stop taking it after a few months. In the long run, it can cause gastrointestinal problems.

Finally, meat replacements also are a plant-based source of protein. At the supermarket, you will find many types of veggie burgers, vegetarian steaks, and meatballs, not only made with soy protein, but also with lentils and chickpeas, which are very tasty!

Following these tips will surely increase your protein intake and will help you revitalize your metabolism.

Another tip you've probably heard before is to use spices. The latter help burn energy and give an additional boost to the metabolism.

There are different kinds of spices that you can choose from, such as turmeric, curry, paprika, etc. Herbs and spices will not only help you cook tastier dishes, but that they will also stimulate your metabolism.

The last piece of advice I want to give you is to take care of your gut. Often what stands behind a sleeping metabolism is a sleeping gut. The bowel is the gateway to our body for energy and nutrients, and it is vital to take care of it. How can you do this? Consume plenty of fiber by eating whole grains rather than refined ones, as well as generous doses of vegetables and legumes. Make sure to have a portion of vegetables at each meal and add them to all the dishes you cook, whether they are meat-, fish-, or (whole) grain-based.

Drinking a lot of water is essential for gut health. I will explain you how you can consume more water in the chapter that describes the three steps to lose weight. Another smart choice is to avoid foods with added sugars such as desserts and sugary drinks, because they are poisons for the gut. Intestinal bacteria, especially bad ones, are particularly greedy of sugar and they can cause flatulence and bloating. Therefore, stay away from added sugars as much as possible.

Take probiotics. The probiotics that I recommend contain both *Lactobacilli* and *Bifidobacteria*. In addition to having both the latter two species, the ideal probiotic should contain more than 10 billion bacterial cells. Many products on the market do not follow these two rules. You will often have to combine two products or two capsules of the same probiotic to get both species of bacteria and a sufficient number of cells.

To conclude this chapter, let's recap the four tips I just gave you: increase lean mass with exercise, get enough protein, use spices in the kitchen, and take care of your gut. If you follow these four simple rules, you will see that your metabolism will finally start working again.

LOSE WEIGHT IN 3 STEPS

"Do you know the TV show "My 600-lb life?" It tells the stories of many people who have severe eating problems (typically a mix of malnutrition, thyroid problems, and psychological problems), who try to lose weight and regain self-esteem and control over their lives. The doctor who follows them, Dr. Nowzaradan, promises to carry out a gastric bypass surgery that can allow them to regain control of their lives, but on one condition: a significant weight loss over a short period of time, which is also a test of their willpower.

Some patients succeed in this feat, while others fail. What impressed me about the program are the protagonists' stories and their determination to change their lives. I remember a man who ate only McDonald's fried chicken, with disastrous results for his health, and a woman who only ate ice cream. These two people were able to lose a lot of weight in a short time.

You won't have to do the same, you are not in that condition, but it is possible to lose weight quickly in a few steps, without energy shakes and phantom supplements. I'm not Dr. Nowzaradan, but I have my tricks, too…Since you bought this book, I guess you have already made several attempts to lose weight over the past years. It's likely you have been exercising every day for several hours with the hope of being able to fit into a smaller clothing size or to be able to finally wear that swimsuit you like so much. Maybe you have been eating smaller and smaller portions, or you stopped eating foods rich in carbohydrates or fats in hopes of losing weight and feeling better.

If you have tried any kind of diet, fasting, extreme exercise, or any other way to lose weight, but your scale always shows the same number or more, you have probably ignored the simplest solution to your problem. The latter is to eat adequate portions of healthy foods that give your body what it needs.

Many people think they need to take drastic action to lose weight. And they are generally surprised to find that there are only three simple steps one needs to do to lose the excess weight and never put it back on.

After all, the diet industry speculates by encouraging diet pills to lose weight or switch to an unhealthy diet. The companies promoting weight loss programs make a lot of money. But the fact is, the weight loss they suggest is only temporary, which means that after a while, your weight will go back to where it was, prompting a new search for solutions that will lead to no results. Those who do so only waste time and money.

I believe that you can and should lose weight differently. When you treat your body with respect, which means not making it feel deprived or without using drastic measures, you will naturally return to your desired weight.

Three simple steps to lose weight

The three steps you need to do to lose weight and never put it back on are steps that respect your body. These are easy actions to take once you know which they are.

The human body senses when we take care of it; therefore, it will take care of us in return. If you feed yourself in a way that keeps you well hydrated, your body will regain its natural balance, and you will gain health.

There is no need to starve or do grueling exercises to lose weight. You simply need to do these three things: maintain an adequate level of satiety, make good healthy food choices, and have enough water in your body to get your body back to working optimally.

My weight loss strategy doesn't focus on drastic calorie restriction. I favor a slight reduction in calories, but there are other important things to consider. Weight loss occurs when you consume less calories than what you would normally consume. Calories from certain foods are associated with many essential nutrients. I've seen hundreds of people lose weight without feeling deprived. These people have learned to choose foods that have a positive influence on their body function. They found out which foods to avoid because they don't provide nutrition to the body. To avoid these foods is a considerable step toward weight loss. When the body gets what it needs, it functions better, the weight remains stable, and food cravings disappear.

I don't believe in extreme diets. Following the Mediterranean diet rules is the best way to lose weight and no longer gain any extra weight. I came to this conclusion after many years of research and focused study on this healthy way of eating.

Now that you know a little more about my approach to weight loss let's get into the three steps you need to take to lose weight and never put it back on.

Increase satiety

The first step to losing weight without exercising or eating a bland diet is to increase satiety with healthy foods in sufficient quantities that will make you feel full. Follow this step at each meal, including breakfast and snacks.

When you choose the right foods and eat them in quantities that satisfy our body, the latter will feel satisfied and will not require more food until the next meal. Most of the time, when you eat foods that meet the body's needs for protein, complex carbohydrates, fiber, and healthy fats to the point of satiety, you don't feel the desire for more food and you do not overeat.

Our body's satiety system is quite brilliant. When we pay attention to it, when we learn to notice when our stomach is asking for food and signals that it is full, we will naturally eat what is necessary for our nourishment. When you are eating, notice your real feeling of hunger and natural sense of fullness, you are acting mindfully, and you will only be taking in the calories you need without putting on extra pounds. A key strategy for losing weight is to listen to your body.

Whenever you think you're hungry, ask yourself, do I just want to eat because it's lunch or dinner time? Instead think, is my hunger real, or do I just need some water? Consider if you are bored and looking for the pleasure of food. When your hunger is real, your stomach starts rumbling, and it will feel empty. The rumbling of hunger is not just a digestive sound. It is a real feeling of emptiness in your stomach. You don't need to eat any food until you have this sensation, which signals it is time to eat. If you're wondering if your hunger is real, try to distract yourself. Go for a walk, do your chores, read, or do anything else. If you can't focus on things to do because your stomach keeps rumbling, then you are hungry and need food. Be careful not to eat without paying attention to what you do.

A key thing to remember when it comes to satiety is that some foods satisfy us, and others don't. Some foods, such as those made with refined flour or lots of junk ingredients, don't have enough nutrients to give you the satiety you need. Of course, they physically fill the stomach. But they don't contain the necessary vitamins, minerals, protein, carbohydrates, fiber, and healthy fats to give our body the nutrition and energy it needs. Therefore, even if you have just eaten a big meal, you'll soon be hungry again.

So, how do we provide our body with what it needs to feel satisfied? How can we make sure that our body has the nutrients it needs to function and not crave the wrong foods? We make sure that our meals contain protein, complex carbohydrates, fiber, and healthy fats. We pay attention that there are not too many sugars or refined flour in them.

It's best for a healthy diet if you use plant-based foods, whole foods high in protein, complex carbohydrates, fiber, and heart-healthy fats. These are foods of the Mediterranean diet that include plant origin elements such as fruit, vegetables, nuts, seeds, and legumes. These foods contain essential nutrients that the body needs to increase satiety and function properly.

Obviously, you will feel hunger signals a few hours after each meal. When you sense these hunger signals, eat a meal that provides the essential nutrients I mentioned above. Your meal should contain the foods I mentioned earlier (legumes, vegetables, etc.), an easy thing to do when you have some recipes to eat them (this book contains several useful and tasty recipes). As you begin your journey to satiety, you will see your body respond positively to the food you are giving it. You will undoubtedly be happy to prove that the wise choice of choosing nutritious calories means that you don't have to eat too many. You will see how full and satisfied your stomach feels, and you will notice that you will lose weight, even when it seems like you are eating more. Your body has begun to regulate itself. You will be thrilled!

I'm going to give you some real examples of meals you can eat to feel full: first I have to tell you that it's important to eat slowly to give your body enough time to process what you are eating. Don't gorge yourself by throwing food down your throat. If you do this, you will find yourself eating faster than your body can digest, and you will overeat. A good rule of thumb is to keep up with the slowest person at the dinner table. If no one is eating slowly, you can be the slowest eater. As you eat, taste each bite, notice its flavor and texture, and chew just enough to aid digestion.

Start with a healthy, filling breakfast

Breakfast can really make a big difference when it comes to satiety. I recommend having a breakfast that offers a combination of protein, complex carbohydrates, fiber, and healthy fats. This breakfast type can simply consist of a bowl of vegetable milk, or unsweetened yogurt, along with fresh fruit and muesli, also without added sugar. Depending on how you prepare your yogurt, you may be able to make it through lunchtime without snacks. Otherwise, if you can't, it's okay anyway. Based on what your yogurt-based breakfast is like, your choice of fruit and granola will help determine if you'll need a small snack before lunch. When you eat yogurt, consume it slowly and pay attention to your body's reaction. Only eat until you feel a sense of fullness. I've also noticed that Greek yogurt makes you feel fuller than other yogurts. But beware that it is also rich in fats!

When choosing yogurt, opt for one that doesn't contain a lot of sugar. Choose a natural yogurt that has no artificial colors or flavors. When selecting fruit to put in your yogurt, use fruit like cantaloupe, whose watery texture makes the yogurt less thick in the mouth, which sometimes means you don't need to eat as much of it to feel full.

The muesli you choose must contain whole grains, nuts, dried fruit, and zero added sugars. The whole grains and nuts in granola will give you all the nutrients you need to energize your body. Many people are reluctant to eat nuts (walnuts, almonds, etc.) because they think it is caloric and fat. Although this is true, it does not mean you need to stay away from nuts. Add some to your muesli or yogurt. Nuts are not a problem for weight loss because you are only eating a moderate amount. Your body needs the protein, fiber, complex carbohydrates, and healthy fats that they provide. Nuts are suitable for children and teenagers as well. They contain fat, but it's healthy fat which doesn't make you gain weight unless you eat more than your body needs.

As a general guideline, I recommend that women keep their daily dried fruit intake between 20 and 30 grams. Men can eat about 30 to 40 grams of nuts per day.

Start other meals with a filling salad

Every time you start a meal, I suggest you start with a large vegetable salad. Chances are you'll feel full right after eating it, which means your stomach won't have any other room for tons of different foods. To start each meal with a salad is a great way to make sure you've eaten your veggies and refrain from filling your belly with much more caloric foods.

When preparing your salad, you need to make sure it contains vegetables other than plain lettuce. Add crunchy vegetables like peppers or fennel. You should also include some healthy protein and fiber sources such as seeds, pine nuts, raisins, goji berries, sliced almonds, chopped walnuts, sesame seeds, hard vegetables like celery and carrots. These ingredients stimulate satiety by encouraging chewing, which gives your body time to process the calories you eat.

Replace high-glycemic carbohydrates with healthy fats

The second step to losing weight and maintaining it is to reduce your high-glycemic carbohydrate intake (especially foods rich in sugar), making smart substitutions. I believe you should consume a limited amount of carbohydrates from refined sources such as white bread, non-wholegrain pasta, rice, and desserts. Other complex carbohydrates, such as whole meal bread and pasta, should be consumed in moderation so that there is room in the diet for other important protein, fat, and high-fiber foods such as legumes, seeds, and nuts.

There are a few tricks you can use to reduce your carb intake. You can halve the amount of pasta, bread, and rice you usually consume and eat more vegetables. I always provide my customers with amazing recipes full of tasty vegetables, and you will find many in this book as well. After cooking their meals with my recipes, many admit that vegetables are now their favorite foods.

As for pasta, bread, and rice, make sure you don't eat more than 50-80 grams per meal. It helps to vary your carbohydrate sources if you are in the habit of only ever eating rice and wheat. A good idea is to have some quinoa. Quinoa is a healthy source of carbohydrates and protein and is excellent for making salads, soups, and stews. My recipes will show you how to use this food to meet your carbohydrate needs adequately.

Another way you can moderately reduce your carbohydrate intake is to replace half of your ration of pasta, bread, and rice with legumes rich in protein and fat from plant foods. Legumes are excellent sources of protein and are essential sources of fiber. They make an ideal complement to the carbohydrate-rich foods with which you should consume them. It is good to replace some of the carbohydrate-rich foods with foods that are high in fat that are good for the heart, such as nuts, seeds, and avocados. Doing so will give your body that healthy balance of nutrients it needs to function correctly.

Drink smart

Now is the time to talk about my third move to lose weight. The third move I suggest to anyone who wants to lose weight and maintain it is to drink wisely. To lose weight, you need to drink more fluids; in particular, it is necessary to drink healthy liquids such as water. Take away the drinks that do not help you.

Many people don't drink enough, despite water being essential to lose weight. Instead, everyone should drink at least eight glasses of water every day. To make it easier, I recommend keeping a bottle of water on your desk if you work in an office. Alternatively, take it with you wherever you go during the day.

Water is essential for the proper functioning of the body. For our digestive and immune system, and every other system in our body to function correctly, we need to stay hydrated. Hydration allows for proper digestion of the nutrients you get from food. If you drink enough water, your body will feel satisfied and will not need more food.

I recommend that you introduce some daily routines. Drink one glass in the morning and one in the evening, drink herbal teas in the afternoon or the evening, and drink with meals. It is not true that water with meals is counter indicated. You can also use lemon or lime juice to add flavor. Take a sip every time you approach the sink to brush your teeth, or wash the dishes, and keep a bottle of water handy: in the car if you travel a lot or on your desk if you work in the office. You can also install an app on your mobile that reminds you when you need to drink.

While pure water is essential for proper body function, you can help your body get enough water through herbal teas and fruit as well. There are many on the market right now that are very flavorful. The important thing is not to add sugar.

Limit your alcohol consumption to maximum one drink per day. When choosing alcoholic beverages, avoid those with added sugar, as is the case with many cocktails, especially non-alcoholic ones. Try the non-alcoholic beer substitutes. On the market there are also excellent quality and good tasting ones.

There are a couple of final points I would like to mention. The first is that a moderate amount of fruit and vegetable juice every day can help your body remain hydrated. Fruits and vegetables naturally contain water, as does their juice. Another point to remember is that fruit and vegetable-based smoothies are excellent choices for light meals and snacks. Smoothies contain whole fruit or vegetables, which means you'll get protein and carbohydrates.

In conclusion

And so that's it. These are the three steps to lose weight easily, without depriving yourself of anything, and without excessive effort:

1. Increase the level of satiety
2. Replace a portion of refined carbohydrates with healthy fats
3. Drink smart

To sum it up, losing wight and not regaining it back for a long time is easy when you increase your satiety and choose nutrient-rich foods to eat only when your hunger is real. Reduce your consumption of refined foods that are a source of fast carbohydrates, replacing them with foods rich in healthy fats. To lose weight, you need to pay attention to your fluid intake by drinking adequate water and cutting out unhealthy drinks. This last step is crucial for weight loss and maintenance. You need to drink lots of water.

THREE SECRETS FOR INTRODUCING HEALTHY ROUTINES INTO YOUR DAILY LIFE

I am a very organized person, and over time I have established "routines" that I perform daily without even thinking about it. They're part of me now, and I feel weird if I don't do them every day. Introducing routines is a beneficial strategy for losing weight and having a better life, such as doing cardio exercises every day, drinking water and herbal tea before bed, or eating fruit in between meals.

Some Olympic fame athletes have some very interesting habits, which they have incorporated into their lives which can lead to excellent results. For example, diver Kassidy Cook has added a very special practice to her training routine: the night before the competition, she takes a bath in a tub filled with ice. It is not a superstitious ritual, but it has a specific purpose: to rest the legs' tissues and strengthen them to be ready to jump the next day again.

I don't mean that you have to take an ice bath but try to make time for your body to rest. Rest doesn't just happen when you sleep. It is necessary to disconnect during the day. We are not machines.

The great tennis player Djokovic has an exciting morning routine: a glass of water at room temperature, then honey, muesli for breakfast, nuts, seeds, coconut oil, and milk. It is a breakfast designed by its athletic trainers to maximize its performance. Together we can work out a meal plan that fits your needs, even if you don't have to win Wimbledon!

Usain Bolt, the fastest man globally, has a rigorous training regimen and a diet tailored to his needs. However, what makes the difference is the quality of his sleep. Bolt sleeps a lot, always going to sleep at the usual time. In this way, your body can regenerate and rest.

I will never stop stressing the importance of sleep. Go to bed at the same time every night, except for a few occasions.

Even the Juventus champion, Cristiano Ronaldo, is a fanatic lover of his body. Ronaldo eats practically every two hours, with meals designed to maximize his athletic performance, has a sleep schedule tailored to his needs (a series of broken naps), and never misses a training session, even late at night.

You don't necessarily have to follow this lifestyle, but you must have the same determination. If you change your diet or start exercising consistently, stick to the new routine you've chosen.

These are sports champions, but what are the three routines that I can suggest to you and put into practice immediately?

Here they are!

One of the most important things if you want to lose weight or simply eat healthier is to make sure that certain good habits become a routine. To establish new practices is easier said than done, which is why in this chapter, I want to give you some tips to transform new healthy habits into routines that will gradually and steadily enter your life.

Self-discipline is fundamental because being more disciplined helps you practice new, healthy habits more easily. Remember that it takes time before you can make a new habit automatic, so don't be discouraged because it takes at least a couple of months for a new practice to become a routine. In time, you will surely succeed.

So let's start with some tips for introducing healthy routines into your daily life. My first piece of advice is to decide a goal. An example could be to have a "smart" salad at the beginning of each meal, as I wrote in the previous chapter. This goal is specific because it refers to starting each meal with a salad that has the characteristics. An example of a non-specific goal would have been to increase vegetable consumption, which could mean anything between one leaf of lettuce per day to eating one pound of vegetables per hour! It's always advisable to be as specific as possible when setting a new goal so that it will be easier to evaluate your progress. You don't need to over-do it at the beginning, you could start by introducing this new habit two to three times a week and gradually increase each week until you get to do it every day.

My first tip to increase your self-discipline is, therefore, to set a specific goal and achieve it gradually.

The second tip I have for you is to come up with an action plan. Your resolutions will never come true unless you have a plan to put them into practice. Let's go back to the example of the salad. You have to organize yourself to buy, for example, the vegetable box every week as well as nuts, pine nuts, seeds, in a nutshell, all the ingredients I've mentioned in the previous chapter.

Next, you need to set a day of the week when you know you have enough time to go to the supermarket and do your grocery shopping. Go shopping with a list of what you need to buy, which makes things easier and reduces the probability to buy foods you should avoid. If you already know that you won't have time every week to go out and buy fresh vegetables, you can arrange to have a crane of vegetables sent directly to your address every week. Alternatively, you can ask someone else to go shopping for you: a family member, a relative, or a friend, for instance. Perhaps, you can also agree with this person that you are going shopping for that both of you take turns every week. Perfect, now you have a plan in place.

Here is my third tip, which is very important: anticipate any obstacles that can make it difficult for you to put your new plan into practice. Always referring to the example of the salad bar, we said that you need to organize your weekly grocery shopping or find someone else who can do this for you. It will undoubtedly happen that something will go wrong; for example, you will not have time a particular week to go shopping and end up without the ingredients you need to prepare your salad. Make sure you have a "Plan B" that will help you fix this potential pitfall. For instance, know which friend you can ask for a favor at the last minute and make sure you can quickly send him/her the list of foods you want to buy.

In summary:

- set a specific goal to be achieved gradually
- prepare yourself with an action plan
- prepare a plan B in case something goes wrong

You will see that you will find it easier to introduce new and healthy routines into your daily life.

Remember: better set yourself a specific, measurable, and easily achievable goal within a certain time frame. The table below gives some examples of specific and quantifiable objectives and suggestions for an action plan and alternatives in case of problems.

Every time the new habit has finally entered your daily life as a routine, you can give yourself a new goal and equip yourself with an action plan. In the following tables I have listed a series of examples of goals, action plans and plan B's.

Specific goal	Action plan	Plan B
Drink an extra half-liter of water per day (3-4 glasses more).	Set an alarm to remind you to drink water.	Install an app with notifications visible even with the ringer off.
Reduce your pasta portions by 20%.	Weigh the amount you consume and recalculate the weight reduced by 20%.	If you're tired of weighing, calculate the number of servings per pack of pasta and mark the box each time you consume it.
Start using aromas in the bedroom to get a better night's sleep.	Order aromas online to spray on the pillow in the evening (for example, valerian), calculate how long it will take you to finish the product, and mark in your diary when it's time to repurchase.	Order two at a time, make a note in your diary, so you don't forget about the next orders.
Get your blood tests done every year.	Choose a date that is easy for you to remember and mark it on your calendar. Keep a list on your computer with the exams to check. Find a lab to take the tests.	You may not be able to take the exams in case of an unexpected event on the day you marked in your diary. Put a second note in your diary a week later, which you remember taking your exams.

THREE TIPS TO IMPROVE YOUR SELF-DISCIPLINE

Do you know Warren Buffet?

He is an American investor, one of the richest men globally, revered by generations of traders. His strategies are taught in economic faculties, and his every action can determine the success or failure of companies and even nations. This man has incredible power in his hands, and he is aware of it. But he has never been given anything in his life; instead, he has earned every single penny with passion, study, and self-discipline.

What does his self-discipline consist of?

It's very simple. Buffet carefully studies the stock market and applies the same method to each company, without ever making exceptions without relying on instinct. Buffet is used to handling large sums of money. He knows that people can deceive you, but numbers cannot.

Warren never changes his way of working, and he still studies the market carefully before doing any investment, even today at an age where he could retire and with so much money that he doesn't know how to spend it.

Why am I telling you about this man? It's simple: Buffet is a genius, but he has always had great discipline, he has a system in place to examine the stock market, he never takes shortcuts, and never makes mistakes. Without his self-control, he would surely have earned less and lost money on reckless investments.

The moral of the story is very simple: if you don't have discipline, you can have a lot of talent and ambitious goals, but you will never achieve them.

How many times have you repeated, or thought about, this sentence? *I can't get anything done because I don't have enough self-determination.* Probably too many. Think about your countless attempts to lose weight and change your lifestyle: do you think you would obtain better results if you could just increase your self-discipline level by a little? The answer to this question is probably yes. But then, how can you be more disciplined when trying to achieve your goal to lose weight? The tips that I am about to give you and which I consider essential to improve your self-determination and self-discipline, are practical and easy to apply in everyday life as usual.

Advice n. 1: Remove all temptations. If your goal is to eat less dessert, get fewer calories and fewer refined carbohydrates in your diet, why do you keep this type of food in your pantry? The most common excuse is that there are children in the house, and they want to eat something sweet every day. Maybe sugar is healthy for them? Get your kids used to more natural sweet flavors from an early age, try recipes for desserts that are sweetened with fruit, for instance. Stop buying sweet foods and eliminate all the foods you don't want to eat from your home such as refined grains, sugary drinks, or alcohol. Don't worry. You will have the opportunity to taste some sweets and a glass of wine from time to time, for instance when you are invited to a celebratory dinner party. When you get rid of "fattening" foods and drinks from your home, it is a good idea to replace these temptations with healthy foods, such as fresh and dried fruit, nuts, or coconut; flavored water and herbal teas can replace sweet drinks and alcohol. Get organized so that you can go shopping for these foods regularly, this way you'll always have these foods on hand and will stay away from the most harmful temptations. Also, when you go to the supermarket, don't walk through the department where they keep all the snacks, desserts, and spirits you like. Especially sodas. Stay away and avoid temptations even on these occasions. Always go shopping with a full stomach.

Think in terms of the temptations you encounter when you go to work or when you bring your children to school, like that pastry shop on the way to work that always has a rich showcase of sweet treats and the pizza shop that sells by the slice. These are all temptations to avoid. Study your daily path to work and think how you can get there walking through streets that do not have too many tempting shops. Who knows, maybe you will even be able to walk a bit more. If you can't avoid walking in front of a tempting store, then walk on the opposite sidewalk.

Another good idea is to regularly shop at organic, healthy shops and restaurants which is a great way to expose yourself to more beneficial foods. Unfortunately, there are also many sweets in organic shops, but maybe you will find a shop that also sells many other healthier food products. The concept is to find more moments in which you expose yourself to more health-promoting environments instead of a supermarket whose shelves overflow with junk and processed food, or a pizza bar that sells a thousand different types of pizzas. Wisely choose the places where you spend your time, so that eating healthier will become easier. The same principle also applies to the people with whom you spend most of your time. Expose yourself to people that live healthily. You can use Meetup.com to search for groups of people who go walking together or who promote a philosophy of healthy living and eating. You will probably meet many vegetarians and maybe even vegans but, even if you don't belong to these categories, why not broaden your horizons?

Advice n. 2. It may seem counterintuitive to you, but I strongly suggest that you enjoy some cheat meals every now and then. I believe it is essential that you reward yourself occasionally, and you can do this without having negative consequences on your weight. I always recommend a cheat meal every week so that you can eat your favorite dish (for me it's pizza) and an extra one every month. Going to a restaurant with your friends does not need to be considered a cheat meal if you choose fish or another protein and order a large bowl of salad and a piece of fruit.

The bottom line is that you can make exceptions from time to time; from a psychological perspective, to give yourself permission to indulge once in a while puts you in a position to have greater self-discipline. No one can resist to all temptations forever you need to let it go sometimes. You know that you can even indulge in a few snags at regular intervals, your sacrifices to lose weight will appear less difficult.

Despite having planned your cheat meals and even though once a week you have your favorite meal. There may be times when you might still not be able to control yourself. You will indulge in a lot of sweets, or you will eat much more than usual, and with little self-control. This usually happens when your stress levels are too high, your commitments have amassed, and you have lost control of your life and, consequently, your diet. What can you do? Learn to forgive yourself, otherwise you will never be able to gain back control of your life and work in a more disciplined manner to a healthy lifestyle.

Be prepared for the fact that there will be times when you will not be able to follow a healthy lifestyle because your commitments will be too looming or because your personal problems will take up all the space in your life and your thoughts. Just remember that a period of weakness is not the end of the world. "To err is human," someone said, and without guilt, you can get back "on the right path" and resume a healthier lifestyle as soon as your life gets back to normal, or as soon as you find the way to adapt your routines to your new situation.

Speaking instead of "non-edible treats," let me remind you that food is not the only reward that exists on planet earth. You can treat yourself by purchasing something you like, or by allowing yourself an extra hour of free time every week for cultivating your passions. When your brain asks for food, it is often merely a signal that you need comfort. Food is simply the quickest way to comfort yourself. Find other solutions. From time to time, you might even indulge in a "crazy" period and go against all the rules you set for yourself and forget your schedule by living life in a more relaxed way for a while. Be careful not to lose your job, though!

Advice n. 3 Concerns of being more "mindful," that is, more conscientious and aware of what you do. You cannot be a self-disciplined person if you have no self-awareness. It is simply impossible! In particular, being more "mindful" when you eat means appreciating food better, noticing and admiring the colors of the food you have on your plate before you put it into your mouth. It means taking time to smell the scent of a dish before tasting it. In a few words, eating mindfully means extending the pleasure of eating to the senses other than your taste. One way to be more mindful is to pay more attention to what you are buying. When you go to the supermarket, stop and read the labels and compare different products with each other. Choose those that do not contain added sugars and additives. Read, document yourself on reputable sites (such as those of health authorities) and avoid trendy nutritionists' advice. Buy books on diet and health written by reputable authors. Take a healthy cooking class and learn how to prepare tasty dishes with simple and genuine ingredients. A disciplined person is, above all, a determined and informed person.

In this chapter, I wrote about self-discipline, the importance of rewarding yourself and finding moments to relax. In the next chapter, I would like to address the theme of holidays, a moment in which we often let ourselves go a little too much with results that are also quite devastating. A bit like what happened to Mr. F.

PREVENTING WEIGHT GAIN ON VACATION

I was in my office with Mr. F, a client of mine for a few months who had achieved excellent results. His diet had improved a lot, and his body had shown remarkable progress. But Mr. F was telling me that for the upcoming three weeks, he would not eat properly.

"For what reason?" I asked.

"Every year, I take three weeks of vacation and I go to Cuba to regenerate myself. I fear that I will not be able to follow your advice while I'm there. You know how it is, you relax, you want to have fun, some excess ... "

"Well, we have already achieved excellent results; it is absolutely okay to take a break and relax a little; it won't be the end of the world. You know what to eat and what not to. Just keep in mind the basic rules I taught you, and you will have no problems," I replied. Up to that moment, Mr. F had benefited from my indications. There were no reasons to think that his holiday could represent a threat for any specific reasons.But I was wrong. And by a lot.

Mr. F came back to me after spending three weeks in Cuba. He was tanned, very tanned.

And heavier. Much heavier.

I'm not exaggerating. Mr. F had gained twenty kg in three weeks!

All good intentions had vanished like fog in the hot Caribbean sun; parties, a lot of food and alcohol, had destroyed months of work. It looked like he had been locked up in a candy shop for three weeks. It was the only explanation I could imagine.

"Doc, I let myself go. But just a little," he told me.

That's why when a client tells me they're going on vacation I feel a cold shiver run down my spine. Fortunately, not everyone is like Mr. F, and holidays usually do not represent a huge hurdle.

This chapter is dedicated to the time when you allow yourself to relax a bit. Perhaps on a beautiful beach, or when you are joyful, going overboard with food and drinks while you go out every night. When you are on vacation, you don't worry much about what (or how much) you eat. However, at a certain point, you might think: Oh, my goodness will I go home twenty-pounds heavier?

Let's see how you can enjoy your much-deserved holidays without spoiling them with negative thoughts about going home with a little extra baggage (and not in your suitcase)!

Every year around September, an avalanche of "repentant" vacationers visit my office. No surprise, right? Another interesting phenomenon is those clients who cancel their follow-up appointment with me because they went up in weight, and they do not want me to see them before getting back into shape.I know that you want to relax on vacation and you certainly don't want to think about diets and scales. Maybe you've been on a diet all year and want to let it go a little during summertime, or at least when you get the chance to go on a trip somewhere. No problem, I totally understand that very well. However, I can teach you some tricks that will help you limit the potential damage that your holidays can do to your shape and help you keep your weight at bay even when you are on vacation.

The first trick I want to teach you is to weigh yourself every other day. It may seem strange that I am telling you to weigh yourself when you are on vacation. However, keeping your body weight under control will enable you to limit yourself a little in your food choices, perhaps avoiding excessive consumption of high-calorie foods and being smart about the treats you choose. Many studies confirm that weighing regularly helps keep weight under control to avoid excessive weight gain. A valid and even more practical alternative is to use a tape measure on your waist every second or third day.

Along the lines of the concept of self-control, here are other exciting ideas for you:

What better way to check your body shape than to try on clothes in a boutique? Holidays are the ideal time to visit new shops and outlets. Try on clothes of your size and see if they still "fit" you. If they don't, it will mean that you have gained weight.   Ask your travel companions to keep an eye on you and to warn you if you are going overboard with processed food, desserts, or alcoholic drinks. You have to choose travel companions who are not binge eaters or drinkers, though, otherwise you won't be able to rely on their judgement!Take advantage of the mirrors you find in the hotel to check that your physical shape has remained unchanged. To make good use of mirrors is a quick and practical way to do a little check-up from time to time. Better not to do it every day because otherwise, the eye will gradually get used to your new "shape." A check every three to four days is more than enough.   My second piece of advice is to exceed with cunning. When you are on vacation, you want to go to a good restaurant with your friends and have fun. I'm not the kind of person who says you should not do this. At the end of the day, I do it, too. However, if you have to do a sin, do it with cunning. Have a cheat meal when it's worth it. Choose a good restaurant, check the reviews carefully, and eat something delicious and typical of the place you are visiting. Take the opportunity to discover new dishes and local delicacies instead of bingeing on industrial ice cream that you can find at any petrol station on the planet or eating fast food or prepackaged pizzas that you bought at the supermarket. If you travel abroad, unless you visit remote places, you will always find good restaurants that serve local food where you can taste something new.

When I am on vacation, I usually skip lunch and have breakfast and dinner only. I always book a hotel where breakfast is available as a buffet so that I can choose protein foods (eggs, cheese, yogurt) that will keep me full until dinner. By acting this way, I can keep myself full for the whole day without risking eating while I'm out of the hotel where the choice is usually between an ice cream or other not very "dietetic" foods. However, don't choose a hotel with a buffet breakfast if you already know you will not be able to be selective and you will end up choosing croissants and other unhealthy foods. When I eat in a restaurant, I choose wisely, for example, a fish restaurant. Maintaining control over what you eat is always the key.

Hunt for stunning landscapes or visit nice places at dawn. Sit back and enjoy the view. Flower markets are also a great place to have an "indigestion" of colors and scents, which will make you forget food for a while. Visiting remote but beautiful places is often the best way to enjoy breathtaking landscapes and exercise. Usually, the most enchanting places are also inaccessible by car or public transport and require you to walk a certain distance. Discover the gems that the area where you are staying offers and enjoy the spectacle of nature. Remember to bring water with you, but not too much food. This moment is supposed to help you relax and should not become another excuse to binge!

Tip number three: Be more active. If you spend your entire holiday lying on the beach or at the border of a pool sipping cocktails and beer, you will probably put on a lot of weight. It's okay to spend some time doing nothing, of course, but you can also take a walk in a park or on the seaside a few times every day. Many resorts offer the opportunity to play beach volleyball or tennis. In a nutshell, have fun in an active way. I personally love taking long walks on the beach while listening to good music. It's a great way to recharge my battery which also allows me to concentrate and meditate. The vacation can also become a time for you to come up with new ideas for your work or family. Or maybe an idea for your next destination! Every morning, when you get up, have your breakfast and then go out for a walk for at least half an hour. If you do this every day, it will surely help you not gain weight.

To visit a new city or to go to the mountains are both great opportunities for doing more physical activity while on holiday since you will walk all day. Always beware of too much sedentary lifestyle.

Your holidays also represent the best time to try a new sport; why not take ski, dance, horse riding or tennis lessons? You do not need to become a champion the most important thing is to have fun while you're being physically active. Who knows, maybe you will return home with the desire to continue your new passion.

Holiday resorts often offer the possibility to sign up for gym sessions on the beach which are usually done with music and are very fun. See if you can book a place where they offer this kind of entertainment.

One last tip: When you are on vacation, you want to relax and reward yourself, I know. However, there are other ways to relax than putting your legs under a restaurant table. For instance, why not book a day at the spa? Many holiday resorts have excellent spas or thermal baths where you can relax and get a massage. Enjoy a relaxing day that will improve your mood and forget food for once. And when you're done at the spa, have a nice walk and breathe in some fresh air!

Head massage is a really cool idea, I did this treatment recently and I have enjoyed it a lot. Search the internet and see if you can find someone close to your hotel.

Finally, is there a better way to relax than sleeping? Vacation is the best time to get more sleep. Lack of sleep negatively affects body weight. Release the accumulated stress and get ready for a long rest. Choose quiet, secluded vacation spots, especially if you know you're short of sleep due to stress or busy family commitments.

In the next chapter I will (finally) give you some ideas about healthy cooking. Stay tuned!

Does a "slimming" cuisine exist?

In the next few chapters, I'll offer you many ideas for learning how to cook quickly to lose weight.

I have coached hundreds of people during their weight loss journey, and one of the comments I most often receive is that my recipes are delicious and filling. That's why in this book, I have included several examples from my diet cookbook (which now includes over 300 recipes) that you will find in the last section.

Cooking for weight loss is an activity that requires organization. It is not enough to know how to put together the ingredients you find in the refrigerator, but you need to shop in a smart and organized way so that the right ingredients are never missing in your pantry. It is vital to have a well-organized kitchen so that there is no downtime.

By reading the upcoming chapters, you will learn how to cook healthy foods, such as whole grains, legumes, or fish, and how to enhance their taste and nutritional properties.I will also explain how to use vegetable oils correctly based on the preparations you need to make and how to use aromatic herbs to enhance your dishes' flavors without overusing salt.

My recipes have been a fundamental component of my nutritional coaching programs for years. If you're ready, we can start our cooking journey and discover the principles of a healthy and satiating cuisine!

Shop smart

Before you learn how to cook, you need to learn how to shop strategically. In this chapter, I will teach you some basic principles and ideas for shopping more mindfully and how to go home with fewer calories in your bag.

The first principle of smart spending is to get organized. Make a shopping list and only buy products that are out of stock in your pantry. Focus on healthy ingredients, such as fruit, vegetables, legumes, nuts, fish, and whole grains, but also herbs and spices. Avoid going to the supermarket looking through the shelves for all the things you need, and you will end up buying a lot more foods than necessary. You can save your shopping list on your phone using a common clipboard app, so it will always be ready to use when you need it. Shopping in a strategic and organized way also means knowing the brands and products to prefer; in general, those without added sugars. Make an inventory of the brands that do not add sugar to their products, especially for the "risky" foods such as yogurt, breakfast cereals, pasta sauces, balsamic vinegar, etc. An alternative to shopping at the supermarket is online shopping; nowadays several supermarkets offer home delivery, and you can order directly from their website. You can also sign up to have a box of mixed fruit and vegetables delivered to your address every week. In case this type of service is not available where you live or it costs too much, you can organize yourself by finding a family member or friend who can replace you when you don't have time to go to the supermarket. Remember to give this person a shopping list with the correct brands and products listed.

The second basic principle that you need to follow if you want to do grocery shopping without risks is to avoid dangerous situations. The latter includes going to the supermarket when you are hungry, which will make you buy more than you need or buy high-calorie foods. It is always best to go shopping after lunch or dinner. Likewise, it is preferred not to shop when you are in a hurry; otherwise, you will not be fully aware of what you are buying as you should. Schedule your shopping like any other commitment and put it on your calendar. If you use online calendars (Google, Apple, etc.), you will find your to-do list on all your devices; if you start using a calendar to schedule all your commitments, your life will be more organized in general. Also, once inside the supermarket, avoid departments that expose caloric foods such as sweets, alcohol, and sausages to avoid unnecessary temptations. This simple trick will make you buy far fewer foods and definitely won't make you buy the most gluttonous, calorie-dense foods. Another good idea is to visit organic shops or go to the market to buy fresh, local products.

The third principle that you can apply to shop in a smarter way is to try new types of foods. It is quite common for many people to always buy the same things we do that because shopping is part of our routine and we often go on autopilot. However, nothing forbids to buy new types of grains, legumes, fruits, or vegetables that you have never tried before. You might discover fresh, healthy, and tasty foods that you weren't even aware of. I'm sure you will find something that intrigues you that you have never tasted before. If you usually do your grocery shopping at a small shop or supermarket, try a larger one that offers a wider selection of food products. Foods from other countries can reserve some surprises, such as Ajvar, a tomato, pepper, and eggplant sauce typical of former Yugoslavian countries. When shopping, don't forget to buy aromatic herbs and pick a variety of herbs, such as marjoram, thyme, wild fennel, burnet, borage, dill. The choice is vast. Try something new every week, and you will see how this habit will enrich your cuisine with a lot more flavor.The last rule for mindful shopping that I want to teach you is to focus on the quality and simplicity of what you buy. Always prefer fresh, dry (as in legumes), or frozen (but not pre-cooked) products to processed and canned ones. Freeze-dried products might look healthier than canned ones, but they are often based on cheap and unhealthy ingredients. On the other hand, simplicity translates into buying the ingredients you need to cook your dishes by yourself. If you don't fancy cooking, you can also buy foods that will allow you to prepare dishes that don't need cooking, like salads. To simplify the kitchen procedures, you can equip yourself with an appliance that helps you cook, for example, a slow cooker that will simmer your food, turning them into super tasty dishes.

I am convinced that, as soon as you start applying the above three principles, you will start reducing the number of calories you put into your basket and you will buy foods of higher quality.

The essentials in the pantry for a healthy and tasty diet

In the previous chapter, we discussed how to shop more wisely and consciously. In this chapter, I want to move on to a more practical discussion and help you understand which foods should never be missing in your pantry and on your shopping list. Having all the essential foods for a healthy and tasty diet at your fingertips helps you eat right more often.

I have already mentioned how important it is that you start your day with a satiating breakfast, for instance with plain unsweetened yogurt with muesli, both with no added sugar. Make sure you buy muesli made with whole grains, nuts, and dried fruit, to combine all their nutritional properties. As an alternative to this breakfast, you can always keep whole meal bread and almond butter at home to make small toasts using wholegrain bread. Or again, vegetable milk and sesame seeds to prepare the pudding. The choice is yours!

If you want to eat healthier, you need consume more vegetables and more fruit. I guess you already knew this. Your pantry should always contain a mix of vegetables and fruits of various types (lettuce, carrots, apples, pears, etc.). Season your vegetables with extra virgin olive oil and always keep a bottle of it in the pantry. Sesame or walnut oil can be used for seasoning as well, if you want to vary the flavor. Remember that the both sesame and walnut oil should only be used raw; although olive oil becomes spoilt as well when cooked, it does not produce unhealthy chemicals unless it is eaten at high temperatures. Don't forget to add some seeds to your salad since they contain valuable phytochemicals: sunflower, flax, or hemp seeds. Olives (black or green), as well as capers, will add extra flavor to your salads.

In addition to vegetables, it is crucial that legumes, a valuable vegetable protein source, are never lacking in your house. Make sure you always have chickpeas, beans, lentils, peas, and green beans in the pantry, preferably dried or frozen. A great way to consume more legumes is to make chickpea or lentil hummus. For this preparation, it is necessary to have (in addition to the olive oil we talked about previously) tahini or almond butter, parsley, garlic, and a couple of lemons. A tasty variation involves the addition of a pumpkin puree.

To give more flavor to all your dishes, I always recommend that you have various spices in your pantry, such as pepper, nutmeg, curry, ginger, cumin, and chili powder. Don't forget aromatic herbs like basil, rosemary, oregano, thyme, sage, and bay leaves will allow you to give more flavor to meat and fish dishes.

To sum it up, here is what should never be missing in your pantry: natural yogurt, muesli, mixed vegetables and fruit, vinegar, extra virgin olive oil, seeds, olives, capers, dried or frozen legumes, tahini or almond butter, garlic, lemons, parsley, spices and aromatic herbs of various kinds. Now you can go shopping, if possible, not on an empty stomach!

How to cook faster

Time is a limited resource and if you have a very busy job and a family, chances are the time you have available for cooking your meals is very short, if not almost non-existant! That is why I thought it might be wise to teach you some techniques that you can apply to cook faster, so that you will be able to do it more frequently. Here are a list of tips and ideas:

Optimize the kitchen for speed

Cooking is, in most cases, a pleasant activity. However, sometimes we give up cooking a dish we like because it takes too long to prepare. You may never have thought about it, but you can increase the speed at which you cook just by organizing the cooking zone so that everything you need is within your reach. I have put together eight tips that will guide you in reorganizing your kitchen and allow you to prepare your favorite dishes more quickly. Here they are:

Tip number 1 - Store your pots and pans in the most accessible place in the kitchen. It could be the cupboard that is right in front of your head or, as it happens in many kitchens, or you could have a pull-out drawer for the pots. You can also buy a rake to hang the pots you use most frequently on the wall near the stove.

Tip number 2 - Make sure that the most frequently used utensils are near the stove. It seems trivial, but often looking for pots and utensils takes time. Then place colored and decorative jars on the counter as containers and insert all the utensils you need: ladle, fork, etc. In this case, you can equip yourself with a small rack where you can hang these objects right in front of you.

Tip number 3 - Keep herbs and spices on hand in a cool, dark place near the stove, for example, in a drawer next to the oven. Alternatively, installing a rotating base shelf inside a cabinet (in the US they call it 'lazy Susan') will make them more easily accessible.

Tip number 4 - Prioritize the items in your pantry and refrigerator. Put the ones you use every day in the front and the ones you use less frequently in the back. Always remember to place cooked dishes on the top shelves and raw foods on the bottom. This disposition will avoid cross-contamination between raw and cooked dishes since the latter have a lower microbial load than uncooked foods.

Tip number 5 - Grains, beans, and other dry foods that you use often can be stored in jars on the counter near the cooking area or in view on another kitchen table, but always close to the stove.

Tip number 6 - It is useful to have a basket of onions and garlic close at hand or otherwise keep them in the refrigerator in a visible position, such as the door.

Tip number 7 - Prepare the cooking zone before cooking to avoid unnecessarily prolonging cooking time because you have to continually look for ingredients, pots, and utensils. Get everything you need out at the start of each preparation. Keep a cutting board near the stove. If you need measuring cups, spoons, or bowls, keep them in the drawer at hand.

<u>Tip number 8</u> - Place a waste bowl on the cooking counter to avoid frequent trips to the garbage can.

You have probably already applied some of these tricks in your kitchen, but I am sure that some of them will be new to you. If you follow these few simple rules, you will cook faster and more efficiently, and the final cleaning will be much easier for you. To cook more quickly is just one of the many ways I can teach you to improve your meal preparation and make sure you will cook more often. In the second part of this chapter, you will find many other ideas and tips for cooking healthy and tasty dishes more often.

Techniques to cook more quickly

Before going into the details of each food group's specific cooking techniques, I would like to illustrate some of my fast cooking ideas. You probably work or have a family to look after and don't have a lot of time to cook. That's why I thought I'd give you some ideas to cook faster by avoiding reheating another pre-cooked food or opening another box of canned meat. What follows are ten rules that will make your life in the kitchen a lot easier:

Put hot water in the tea kettle, and it will boil faster than on the stove. Remember to add salt when the water is boiling and not before, as the salted water takes longer to cook.   The raw leaves of spinach, chard, and other vegetables that you eat cooked, can be sautéed with oil and garlic. You may not know, but you can also cook rucola this way; mixed with baby spinach offers a pleasant bittersweet contrast.   Freeze chopped onion, celery, and carrot so that you always have the basis for a good sauté at hand. You can also freeze minced garlic to preserve it longer. In the evening, put the dried legumes in a visible position (perhaps in a milk jug): you will remember more easily to soak them before going to work the next morning, and in the evening, you will cook them more quickly. Buy a pressure cooker and a good microwave. Cooking double portions will allow you to eat another healthy meal the next day. But be careful not to eat twice as much! Divide the two portions before bringing one of them to the table and immediately place the other one into the freezer. Peel the carrots with a potato peeler and slice them *à la julienne* with a grater. These methods will allow you to cook these vegetables much faster than usual with a little oil. Alternatively, once sliced, they will be ready to be seasoned. You can eat zucchini raw, sliced with a grater, did you know? When you buy fish fillets, ask the butcher to cut them into bite-sized pieces so that they are ready to cook like soup. Buy frozen bags of mixed vegetables and legumes: cooked with a little rice, pasta, barley, or quinoa, together with aromatic herbs such as rosemary, they will allow you to prepare an excellent soup quickly.

Save time by freezing cooked vegetables

Storing cooked vegetables in the home freezer allows you to eat mushrooms, aubergines, courgettes, peppers, and many other vegetables or legumes even when you don't have time to go shopping or pick them up in the garden. However, it is useful to know some basic tricks to properly freeze cooked vegetables, to enjoy them at their best once they have thawed. In general, rapid cooking (2 to 5 minutes) is sufficient and prevents the vegetables from becoming mushy once thawed. You can stop cooking by soaking the vegetables in a solution of water and ice. Next, try slicing the vegetables (or cutting them into cubes, rounds, or match sticks) and, above all, drying them well, then placing them in a freezer bag. Freezing dry food will prevent excess ice from forming. In the particular case of spinach, the leaves should rest for a long time in a colander before freezing them to eliminate the water that slowly comes out of the leaves. In the case of grilled vegetables (e.g., peppers), it is better to press them with a fork to remove the cooking water before freezing them. The artichokes must be thoroughly cleaned and soaked in a water and lemon solution before cooking to prevent oxidation. Finally, another excellent idea is to freeze all the soup directly in airtight containers, whether pasta, rice, quinoa, or just vegetables and legumes.

Cook a three-course dinner in thirty minutes

A handy kitchen tool for those who have little time and want to reduce calories is certainly the steamer. Many know it only when it comes to cooking vegetables, but this useful appliance can also cook rice, fish, and meat. Let me explain how you can cook a three-course dinner in record time, thanks to this handy tool. To cook a "sprint" three-course dinner proceed as follows: put some rice and vegetable broth in the upper basket of your steamer, turn it on and let it run for five minutes. As the rice begins to cook, slice some vegetables of different kinds: asparagus, courgettes, and peas, for instance. Place these vegetables in the second basket of your steamer. Wait another five minutes, after which you will add some fish fillets in the lowest basket. Sprinkle your fillet with herbs like rosemary, dill, or sage. Remember to dress it with extra virgin olive oil and, if you like, chopped parsley, lime or lemon juice, or with green sauce. Finally, simmer your rice with a piece of butter and grated parmesan cheese before serving it. If you want, season with extra virgin olive oil and truffle if you love Mediterranean flavors. Alternatively, if you prefer oriental flavors, add curry, soy sauce, or masala. So, your three-course dinner is ready after just thirty minutes. Enjoy your meal!

Other strategies for cooking fast

Before closing this chapter, let me give you a few more ideas to cook fast, so that from now on you will be able to cook more frequently, which will help you gain health over time. Apply one or more of the eight strategies below, and you will see that you will be able to prepare a meal quickly and easily.

Strategy no. 1: preparation is key

Always keep the pantry well-stocked with essential quick-cooking ingredients such as pasta, rice, broth, canned tomatoes, lean meat, frozen fish fillets, frozen vegetables, eggs, dried or canned beans, and extra virgin olive oil.

Strategy no. 2: choose a quick-cooking method

When you need to reduce time in the kitchen, cooking can be the weak point of the whole chain. When you're short on time, such as finishing work late or stuck in traffic, apply one of the following quick cooking methods to cook a quick dinner:

Grilling: ideal for cooking the classic chicken breast or fish fillet. If these foods are frozen, defrost them in the microwave.   Cooking in a pan with a little oil: to sauté the vegetables (perhaps pre-cooked for 3 minutes in the microwave at maximum power) or prepare fried eggs.   Steam cooking: ideal for cooking vegetables or fish, for example. If you do not have the steamer while boiling pasta, rice, or legumes, place a metal colander over the pot and cook combined.   Microwave cooking: even if it does not always produce an excellent result taste wise, it is certainly suitable for all foods, including risotto. Many commercial microwaves come with a cookbook.

Strategy no. 3: be aware of the different cooking times

This strategy is worth more than anything else when you want to cook several dishes simultaneously. Estimate the time needed to prepare each dish and organize each dish's preparation sequence in descending order of preparation time.

Strategy no. 4: grate the vegetables before cooking them

It may seem trivial, but it is not. If you don't want to eat raw vegetables all the time, grate them instead of slicing them, and they will cook much faster.

Strategy no. 5: the thinner it is, the faster it will cook

Complementary to the previous strategy, consider that cutting ingredients into smaller chunks means less time cooking them. When cooking meat, fish, and vegetables, cut everything into small pieces; you will notice a significant decrease in cooking times.

Strategy no. 6: take advantage of the steam from cooking

I mentioned it before but let me repeat it: when you boil something, place a colander with fresh vegetables or fish on top of the pot. Cover with a lid, and the steam will cook other foods quickly. This technique is also ideal for cooking the meal you'll take to work the next day.

Strategy no. 7: precook in the microwave

Pre-cooking the most challenging vegetables in the microwave before actual cooking speeds up cooking times by a great deal. You can try putting some peppers in the microwave for three to five minutes on full power before sautéing them. The microwave pre-cooking also works well with carrots and potatoes to be used later for cooking soups or stews.

Strategy no. 8: buy convenient foods

Adding some ready-made products to the menu can help reduce the time needed to prepare your meals. These can include roast beef prepared in a trusted restaurant or food store or vegetables that the greengrocer sells already chopped or pre-cooked. Avoid processed food, though.

Cooking is more fun when you move smoothly and quickly throughout the entire process. Follow the above simple, quick-cooking rules and prepare your first sprint recipe right away!

How to replace animal protein with vegetable protein

In this chapter, I'll give you all the information you need to cook high-protein foods (such as whole grains, legumes, eggs, and fish) according to the principles I teach in my diet programs.

How to replace animal protein with vegetable protein

To swap animal protein for plant protein is healthy but it's also challenging. Most of my clients have eaten animal protein their entire lives, and many of them do not even know they can get protein from plants as well. As a matter of fact, how many people consider grains a high-protein food? Chances are that very few people know this. If all this sounds familiar, let me give you a couple of ideas to help you swap animal protein with plant-based protein.

Let me start with an example that includes two classic dishes that are animal protein based: a hamburger (which is made of ground meat) and pizza (which contains cheese, and some toppings like salami). The first one can be replaced by a plant-based burger, made with vegetables, lentils, mushrooms, potatoes, and other plant-based foods. Online you can find many recipes to prepare delicious veggie burgers. You can also buy ready-made veggie burgers at your favorite grocery store but check the ingredient list and avoid those that contain sugar, preservatives, or other unhealthy ingredients. There are vegan burgers for all tastes since each type comes with its specific flavor. You can make a great veggie burger at home using lettuce, tomato, tofu, and even with toppings like barbecue sauce or avocado. Place your burger in two slices of whole meal bread and enjoy.Speaking of pizza instead, you can easily skip animal protein by using whole wheat flour, tomato sauce, and vegetable toppings like broccoli, artichokes, onions, mushrooms, or spinach. Add some garlic (if you like), some grated tofu, and maybe some other vegan meat replacements like grilled tempeh slices.

These are just a few examples of how you can replace animal protein with vegetable protein, but the possibilities are manifold, like preparing a smoothie using an unsweetened vegetable milk (rice, almond, soy, etc.) instead of cow's milk.One of the best ways to replace animal protein with vegetable protein is to consume legumes more often. Legumes are plants that have been cultivated since ancient times in the Mediterranean area. These crops originated in the Middle East, where the cultivation of peas, lentils, chickpeas, and vetch was introduced in ancient times. Vetch is more common as animal feed, but nothing prevents you from using it in your salads. Legumes are used during crop rotation because they are able to fix atmospheric nitrogen through rhizobia,[1] allowing the soil to regenerate its nitrogen content. The legumes' seeds are often available dried which have a long shelf life. Some people have digestive trouble when eating legumes. Preparing them in the form of a puree is one way to avoid digestive problems.

As I have already explained before, the combination of legumes and grains provides a complete set of amino acids (the essential components of proteins) to the human body. Protein from grains have a relatively low content in some amino acids, such as lysine and tryptophan which are instead contained in legumes in adequate amounts. On the other hand, the latter lack methionine, a sulfur amino acid found in cereals. Chickpeas, in particular, are a rich source of tryptophan, an essential amino acid that cannot be produced by the human body.

Legumes are not only a source of protein, but also contain many other nutrients: 100 g of chickpeas provide an amount of folate that is almost equal to the recommended daily dose, not to mention many other B vitamins and minerals, including iron. The latter is present in a less soluble form than the iron contained in meat. However, consuming legumes in association with a vitamin C source (such as lemon juice, cabbage, peppers, or tomatoes) increases its solubility, and, consequently, makes it more bioavailable and easier to absorb. These vegetables also provide large amounts of fiber and phytoestrogens, both useful in reducing blood cholesterol levels. Legumes also contain oligosaccharides (such as raffinose and stachyose) that our digestive system cannot process. Therefore, these compounds ferment in the intestine cause an unpleasant-phenomena such as bloating and flatulence. However, a regular legume use will allow your bowel to get used to them and this annoying problem will disappear in time thanks to the help of your gut microflora which feeds itself with these sugars that our body cannot digest. Unfortunately, despite all these critical nutritional qualities, legume consumption is often very low, and it is even demonized by some diet books because of their high content in oxalates and phytates, despite the lack of proof of their negative health consequences.

Which legumes should you choose? It is preferable to use dried or frozen legumes rather than canned ones that contain a lot of salt. Before cooking the dry ones, you will need to soak them in cold water for several hours. Soaking allows to reduce the cooking time and facilitates their digestion. You need to discard the soaking water with fresh water before cooking them, in a volume that must be more than double that occupied by the rehydrated legume. This will help you get rid of some anti-nutrients contained in the legumes. Cooking over low heat (preferably with the addition of bay leaves for flavor) should continue until your legumes reach the desired consistency: a little more "al dente" to use them in salads, well-cooked to prepare a puree. It is best to add salt only after cooking them to avoid hardening of the peel. You can reuse the cooking water to prepare soups and broths.

My best tips for cooking legumes

It always surprises me to see how many people don't know what legumes are. This is because many people refer to them as "beans," but legumes are more than just beans. The category of legumes includes broad bean, pea, chickpea, lentil, soy, and peanut. All legumes are good sources of protein of average biological value. The combination of legumes and grains is an excellent strategy to take the protein equivalent to animal products. Legumes are also an excellent source of soluble fiber and contain a fair amount of essential fats (which cannot be synthesized by the human metabolism) and mineral salts, in particular potassium. Initially, consuming legumes can cause bloating problems, but over time they help maintain good intestinal hygiene. Unfortunately, their vitamin content is significantly reduced by cooking.

Some practical tips:

- Add a bay leaf to the water in which you will boil your legumes. It will give them more flavor and make them more digestible.
- Adding chopped onions and carrots to the cooking water adds even more flavor to your legumes.
- Add the salt only at the end to avoid the hardening of the peel.

Here are some tips to help you speed up the preparation time of legumes.

<u>Tip no. 1</u>: Choose legumes that do not require soaking. Peas and red lentils cook in minutes without soaking. You can also use frozen peas. Defrost them in the microwave, and then sauté them with a bit of olive oil and chopped onion. You can store some sliced onion and garlic in the freezer, perhaps along with chopped carrots and celery.

Tip no. 2: The "quick" soak. It consists of boiling the legumes for two minutes, removing them from the heat, and leaving them in their water for one to four hours. After changing the water, you can cook them for ten to fifteen minutes. All this can be done directly in a pressure cooker to further speed up the time. Alternatively, you can put your legumes in water in the morning before going to work.

Tip no. 3: Use the legumes you prepare over the weekend. On Saturday or Sunday, remember to boil some chickpeas, beans, and peas for more than one serving. Using the pressure cooker will save you time. Once cooked, you can keep them in the freezer or put them in jars with boiling cooking water and seal them. In this case, you will have to keep the jar in the refrigerator and consume the legumes within two to three days of opening it, or in any case, within seven to ten days of preparation. An alternative is to prepare hummus, a chickpea cream, and sesame seed sauce, of which you can find different recipes and variations, and which you can eat with bread.

Tip no. 4: Use the microwave. Put the rinsed legumes in a microwave safe container, cover with cling wrap suitable for the microwave, and prick. Cook on full power for eight to ten minutes or until boiling. Let it sit for one to two hours, stirring occasionally, then drain. If they are still hard, cook or boil them in a pot for a few minutes.

Always remember not to mix different legumes. Cooking times vary. If you are preparing a mixed legume soup, you need to consider their different cooking times, adding the legumes that require longer cooking times first.

Hummus: a creamy way to enjoy legumes

Start by soaking 100 g of dried chickpeas for about twelve hours, boiling them for about half an hour. Then blend the chickpeas adding a few tablespoons of their cooking water a little at a time until you get a cream. To get a creamy hummus, you need to mix the tahini separately with the lemon juice before adding the other ingredients. A generous spoonful of tahini and the juice of half a lemon are enough for 100 g of chickpeas. At this point, add a clove of minced garlic, a generous spoonful of extra virgin olive oil, and a little salt to the mixture of tahini, and lemon juice. Continue to mix until you get a cream. Finally, add the blended chickpeas gradually until the mixture becomes thicker and yellowish. Don't forget to decorate with chopped fresh parsley, and your hummus is ready! Alternatively, you can make hummus with almond butter instead of tahini or lentils instead of chickpeas.

Tuscan cecìna: a gluten-free substitute for bread

To prepare an excellent Tuscan cecìna (which in Liguria is called 'farinata'), preheat the oven to the highest temperature. Put 180 g of chickpea flour in a large bowl; add three tablespoons of extra virgin olive oil, a teaspoon of salt, and, gradually, 600 ml of water. Keep stirring with a whisk to mix the ingredients until you obtain a smooth mixture without lumps. Let it sit until the oven reaches the temperature. Evenly grease a pan of about 26 cm in diameter with oil before pouring the dough. Place in the oven for fifteen to twenty minutes or until a crust forms on the surface. Top with rosemary leaves.

Recipes with legumes

UCCELLETTO BEANS

Ingredients for four people: 800 g of cannellini beans (fresh weight or after soaking), 400 g of tomato pulp, garlic, four tablespoons of extra virgin olive oil, sage, salt, and pepper to taste.

Brown the garlic in the oil. Add the beans and sauté them for a couple of minutes while stirring. Pour the tomato pulp, a little sage, salt, and pepper. Cook over low heat for about half an hour before serving.

CANNELLINI, ZUCCHINI, AND BLACK OLIVE SALAD

Recipe for four people: Mix 200 g of leaf salad of your choice, 300 g of julienned courgettes, 300 g of cannellini beans (cooked weight), ten black olives cut in half, some basil leaves. Season with extra virgin olive oil, and freshly squeezed lemon juice.

ARTICHOKE, CANNELLINI, AND WALNUT SALAD

Recipe for four people: Mix eight stalks of celery cut into rings, 400 g of boiled cannellini beans (weight cooked), eight artichoke hearts cut in half in oil, four tablespoons of walnut kernels, and chives to taste. Season with extra virgin olive oil and freshly squeezed lemon juice.

CHICKPEA, DRIED TOMATO, AND BLACK OLIVE SALAD

Recipe for four people: Mix 200 g of red salad, 400 g of boiled chickpeas (weight cooked), 200 g of dried tomatoes cut into slices, four tablespoons of sliced black olives, four tablespoons of sesame seeds, four tablespoons of hummus (see recipe), chopped parsley. Season with extra virgin olive oil and freshly squeezed lemon juice.

LENTIL SALAD

Recipe for four people: Mix 400 g of boiled black lentils (cooked weight), 200 g of parsnip (or carrot) cut into thin longitudinal sheets with a potato peeler, four tablespoons of dried cranberries, four tablespoons of pine nuts, and chives are a pleasure. Season with extra virgin olive oil and freshly squeezed lemon juice.

SWEET POTATO, LENTIL, AND PISTACHIO SALAD

Recipe for four people: Mix 200 g of mixed leaf salads, 200 g of boiled black lentils (weight when cooked), 400 g of baked or boiled sweet potato cut into chunks, four red onions cut into rings, four tablespoons of pistachios. Season with extra virgin olive oil, and lemon juice.

RED LENTIL CREAM

Ingredients for four people: 800 g of red lentils, two large onions, four cloves, two bay leaves, 50 g of vegetable cream, four tablespoons of extra virgin olive oil (or sesame seeds), ginger flakes, salt and pepper to taste.

Boil the lentils for thirty minutes in a little water together with a bay leaf, and the onion battened with a clove, salt, and pepper. If necessary, add water while cooking, never diluting the lentils too much. After about twenty minutes, add the ginger. Remove from the heat, add the cream, and blend the ingredients with the remaining cooking water. Serve with chopped fresh parsley and a drizzle of raw olive or sesame oil.

SEITAN WITH CURRY

Ingredients for four people: 400 g of sliced seitan, two tablespoons of curry powder, four tablespoons of potato starch, ½ lemon, four tablespoons of extra virgin olive oil, four tablespoons of soy sauce, rosemary, and parsley.

Add the oil, curry, and rosemary to the pan, and mix well. Heat, then add the seitan. Cook the seitan for a couple of minutes on each side, then place it on a plate. Fill half a glass with water, dissolve four tablespoons of starch in it, stirring well, and pour the liquid into a pan. Add the juice of half a lemon and a few drops of soy sauce, to thicken it while stirring. Pour the sauce on the slices of seitan. You can decorate your seitan with lemon slices and parsley.

COUNTRY BEAN SOUP

Ingredients for four people: 300 g of bread, 300 g of fresh broad beans, 300 g of carrots, celery, garlic, wild fennel, four tablespoons of extra virgin olive oil, salt and pepper.

Start by shelling the beans, remove the inner film, and boil them in water. Halfway through cooking (twenty to thirty minutes later) remove half, and mash them with a fork. Put them back in the water, and add some salt and chopped onion, carrot, and celery. After about a quarter of an hour, add some chopped wild fennel, adding more boiling water (if necessary). Carry on cooking for another quarter of an hour. Serve the soup in a deep dish along with slices of chopped bread rubbed with garlic. Season with salt and pepper before serving

PUGLIESE BEAN SOUP

Ingredients for four people: 800 g of broccoli, 400 g of broad beans (weighed after soaking), four tablespoons of extra virgin olive oil, onion, salt and pepper to taste.

Boil the broad beans, after having soaked them for at least twelve hours in water with the onion. Separately, boil the broccoli. Once cooked, drain, and blend the beans. Serve the purée with the boiled broccoli florets; add a pinch of salt and pepper, and sprinkle with raw oil.

LENTIL AND RADICCHIO SOUP

Ingredients for four people: 200 g of red radicchio, half a small onion, 300 g of lentils (cooked weight), four sprigs of fennel, four tablespoons of extra virgin olive oil, salt and pepper to taste.

Cut the radicchio into strips and place it in a saucepan with the boiled lentils, the chopped fennel, and the sliced onion. Cover with water and bring to a boil. Add salt and pepper. Boil for one to two minutes, then blend half of the mixture. Gather the latter with the non-blended part and serve with a teaspoon of oil.

TURMERIC PEA SOUP

Ingredients for four people: 800 g of peas (fresh or thawed weight), 2 kg of fennel, two tablespoons of turmeric, a few mint leaves, four tablespoons of extra virgin olive oil, salt and pepper to taste.

Boil the fennel until tender. Separately, boil the peas. Blend the fennel with their cooking water just enough to obtain a rather liquid cream and put it back on the heat. Add the rest of the ingredients to the fennel cream, bring to a boil for one to two minutes before serving.

MOUNTAIN SOUP

Ingredients for four people: 400 g of lentils, 300 g of chestnuts, 300 g of a mix of carrot, and celery, 100 ml of tomato sauce, one mix of chopped aromatic herbs, a few bay leaves.

Leave the lentils to soak for at least six hours before boiling them in the water together with a bay leaf, other aromatic herbs, peeled and chopped chestnuts, chopped carrot, and celery. Cook until all ingredients have softened. Add the tomato sauce halfway through cooking.

Three ways to make tofu you will love

Tofu is the perfect food to use for plant-based protein instead of animal protein. Many people scrunch their noses when they hear about this food. They have heard it doesn't taste good, or they assume that because it's not common. Or they have tried it and decided they don't particularly like it.

However, tofu is just like any other food, whether vegetable or animal: it can be prepared incorrectly, and therefore won't be as tasty, or you can cook it in a way that it will taste great. Whether you've never tried tofu and didn't think you wanted to try it, whether you've already tasted it and hated it, or you already like it, I think you'll still find these simple recipes enjoyable.

However, a very simple way to prepare tofu is to cut it into slices and place it in a hot pan oiled with a sprinkle of whole salt, and black pepper (and maybe some gomasio). Tofu seasoned this way tastes great on its own or sandwiched between two slices of toasted whole grain bread.

SALTED TOFU WITH TERIYAKI SAUCE

Ingredients for four people: 300 g of tofu, Teriyaki sauce, four tablespoons of extra virgin olive oil.

Drain the tofu and press it with a cloth to release all the water it has absorbed. Cut it into cubes, marinate for fifteen minutes in a bowl where you will have poured a cup of Teriyaki sauce. Sauté it in a pan with a tablespoon of extra virgin olive oil. Run the tofu over the pan, so it doesn't stick to the bottom, and brown it on each side.

TOFU WITH MEXICAN SAUCE

Ingredients for four people: 300 g of tofu, Mexican red sauce, four tablespoons of extra virgin olive oil, four corn tortillas.

Remove the water from the tofu package and press it with a cloth to release all the absorbed water. Cut the tofu into cubes. Marinate the tofu in the Mexican red sauce. Afterward, sauté it again, and add it to corn tortillas. I suggest you garnish with a spoonful of fresh guacamole before enjoying it.

SWEET AND SOUR SALAD WITH TOFU AND DRIED FRUIT

Ingredients for four people: 400 g of leaf salad, 200 g of carrots, 200 g of grilled tofu, 40 g of dried nuts (for example, hazelnuts and almonds), 40 g of goji berries or raisins, two spoons of sesame seeds, four tablespoons of apple vinegar, four tablespoons of mustard, two spoons of extra virgin olive oil, salt and pepper to taste.

Wash and clean the salad and after drying it, roughly break it with your hands. Pour it into a salad bowl. Cut the tofu into cubes after pressing it with a cloth to release the water it has absorbed; grate the carrots and add them to the salad. Pour the Goji berries and sesame seeds into the salad bowl. Make the vinaigrette by emulsifying the oil, apple cider vinegar, salt, pepper, and mustard. Dress the salad with the vinaigrette and serve to the table.

SPELT WITH TOMATOES AND SAUTÉED TOFU

Ingredients for four people: 400 g of spelt, 800 g of cherry tomatoes, 400 g of natural tofu, four tablespoons of extra virgin olive oil, salt, and pepper to taste.

Boil the spelt in salted water for about twenty-five minutes. Meanwhile, press the tofu with a cloth to release the absorbed water. Sear the cherry tomatoes with the diced tofu and the oil in a pan. Drain the spelt, and toss with the other ingredients, including salt and pepper. You can serve immediately or refrigerate for at least a couple of hours if you want to consume it cold.

I hope you fall in love with these recipes. Remember that tofu is an excellent source of protein and is quite filling.

My best tips for cooking grains

If you think about grains, the first thing that probably comes to mind is carbohydrates. These foods are also a source of protein. Grains have been grown by man since the beginning of agriculture. Wheat has long been a staple for Mediterranean populations and is used to produce bread, pasta, bulgur, and couscous. Other popular cereals in southern Europe are rice (grown in Italy, France, and Spain) and corn. Corn flour is the primary ingredient for polenta, a typical dish from Northern Italy.

Whole meal grains should always be your primary choice because they are rich in both fiber and antioxidants. Fiber promotes satiety and slows down starch absorption allowing for a slower glycemic response thanks to a slower rise in blood sugar levels. This phenomenon slows down the return of hunger and prevents pancreas fatigue. On the contrary, starch from refined cereals gets absorbed quickly, especially if consumed without vegetables, provoking a rapid spike in blood sugar levels. The pancreas needs to produce a lot of insulin in a short time, causing blood sugar to drop suddenly. Hunger comes back so quickly, as it is (also) linked to low blood sugar levels. Whole grains also contain phytosterols, folate, magnesium, potassium, selenium, vitamin E, and flavonoids. Unfortunately, wheat processing eliminates the germ, and industrial whole grains often do not contain it because they are simply a mix of refined flour and bran. If you want to eat pasta, choose durum wheat varieties which have a lower glycemic index. Serve it with a vegetable sauce, made with some onion and garlic, as well as extra virgin olive oil.

Some tips for cooking grains

Before using any grains, wash them under current water to remove dust and impurities. When you cook couscous, millet, or buckwheat, toast them before boiling them. The kernels will remain well separated from each other and be more digestible.Cooking times vary from product to product. In any case, cooking can take place in water or broth, and it is also possible to use that by boiling vegetables (cooking water), which is rich in mineral salts. Be careful not to reuse the water in which you soaked your legumes, as the latter could have released some anti-nutrients. You can cook grains in water with a pinch of salt. Cover the pot and cook over gentle heat. When you turn off the heat, mix them with some sautéed vegetables, and let your dish cool for a few minutes before serving. You can turn off the heat halfway when you use earthenware pots because the latter remains hot for a longer time and allows you to simmer your dishes.

Sometimes it may be useful, or necessary, as in the case of rye, to soak the cereal before cooking it to cook your grains in a more homogeneous way and in a shorter time. Some products require special preparation, such as couscous and bulgur. Toast the latter in a little oil, stirring with a wooden spoon, and then pour them into a tureen with boiling salted water, two cups of water for one cup of grains. After about a quarter of an hour, the preparation will have swollen sufficiently. Use cereal flakes to prepare soups, porridges, and creams. You can also mix them with yogurt, perhaps accompanied with fresh or dried fruit.

Recipes with grains

MINT BULGUR

Ingredients for four people: 200 g of bulgur, 1 kg of mixed and sliced vegetables (courgettes, peppers, tomatoes), two tablespoons of pine nuts, two tablespoons of raisins, some mint leaves cut into small pieces, three tablespoons of lemon juice, two tablespoons of extra virgin olive oil.

Boil the bulgur following the directions on the package. Add the other ingredients, sauté, mix, and serve.

PASTA ALLA PIACENTINA

Ingredients for four people: 400 g of pasta, 400 g of fresh beans, 200 g of peeled tomatoes, celery, carrot, onion, garlic, parsley, basil, a tablespoon of extra virgin olive oil, salt, and pepper to taste.

Boil the beans in salted water, with half an onion and chopped celery. While the beans are cooking, prepare a separate sauté of chopped carrot, onion, garlic, and parsley in oil. Let it dry; add the beans (drained), and the peeled tomatoes cut into small pieces. Add salt and pepper. Lower the heat, and let it cook for 5 minutes. Add some chopped fresh basil. Separately, boil the pasta, drain it, and season it with the bean sauce. Sprinkle with pepper and serve.

COUSCOUS ORTOLANO

Ingredients for four people: 350 g of couscous, 1 kg of mixed vegetables, 600 g of ripe tomatoes, white wine, onion, garlic, salt, pepper, and 50 ml of extra virgin olive oil.

Brown the garlic, and onion in half of the oil, add the previously washed and thinly sliced vegetables, salt, pepper, and ripe tomato cut into chunks. Sprinkle with a splash of wine, and let it evaporate. Cook for about twenty-five minutes. Separately, toast the couscous for one to two minutes in the remaining part of the oil then add boiling water in proportions equal to about three times the couscous volume. Let it sit until it swells. Combine the couscous with the vegetables and serve on the table.

MILLET CREAM WITH PUMPKIN AND CROUTONS

Ingredients for four people: 400 grams of millet, 2 kg of pumpkin cut into cubes, four leeks cut into thin slices, vegetable broth, four tablespoons of sesame seed oil, rosemary, four tablespoons of soy sauce, freshly ground white pepper, some croutons.

In a saucepan, sauté a little sesame oil with the leek, chopped rosemary, and diced pumpkin. Cover with the broth, add the millet and cook over low heat for about forty minutes. When cooked, add the soy sauce and white pepper. Reduce everything to a cream using an immersion blender. Serve the millet and pumpkin cream hot with a drizzle of raw oil and some croutons.

WHOLE MEAL FARFALLE WITH BROCCOLI AND PINE NUTS

Ingredients for four people: 400 g of farfalle (a type of pasta), 800 g of broccoli, four to five tablespoons of pine nuts, four tablespoons of extra virgin olive oil, garlic, salt, and pepper to taste.

Lightly brown the garlic in the oil, add the broccoli, and sauté fifteen minutes, occasionally stirring. Separately, boil the pasta in salted water, drain it al dente, and mix it with the broccoli. Garnish with pine nuts, and sprinkle with pepper before serving.

SPELT WITH PESTO AND TOMATOES

Ingredients for four people: 400 g of spelt, 800 g of cherry tomatoes, 50 g of pesto, four tablespoons of extra virgin olive oil, salt, and pepper to taste.

Boil the spelt in salted water for about twenty-five minutes. Meanwhile, cut the cherry tomatoes into four parts, and place them in the colander. Drain the spelt over the cherry tomatoes so that they burn with the cooking water. Stir with the pesto and serve.

BUCKWHEAT WITH MUSHROOMS

Ingredients for four people: 400 g of buckwheat, 800 g of cultivated mushrooms, white onion, white wine, chopped parsley, four tablespoons of extra virgin olive oil, salt, and pepper to taste.

Boil the buckwheat following the directions on the package. Drain it once boiled. Separately, brown the onion in oil, add the finely sliced mushrooms, blend with the wine, add the salt and pepper. Cook for about ten to fifteen minutes. Mix with buckwheat and serve on the table.

BARLEY SALAD WITH TOMATOES

Ingredients for four people: 400 g pearl barley, 400 g red tomatoes, 120 g of drained mushrooms in oil, eight pitted black olives, four tablespoons of extra virgin olive oil, salt, and pepper to taste.

Cook the barley in the pressure cooker for fifteen minutes with 750 ml of water. Wash the tomatoes and dice them. Slice the olives and mushrooms. Drain the barley once cooked and stop cooking by passing it under cold water. Transfer it to a bowl, season it with the oil, and prepare all the previously prepared ingredients. Season with salt, add a little pepper, and, after letting it sit for at least an hour in the refrigerator, serve on the table.

SPELT AND GRILLED VEGETABLE SALAD

Ingredients for four people: 400 g of spelt, 800 g of a mix of vegetables (peppers, courgettes, aubergines, cherry tomatoes), a few basil leaves, four tablespoons of extra virgin olive oil, salt, and pepper to taste.

Wash, clean, and slice the vegetables. Grill them, and season with salt and pepper. Meanwhile, boil the spelt in salted water, following the directions on the package. Drain it and toss with the other vegetables and oil before serving.

QUINOA SALAD

Ingredients for four people: 200 g of quinoa, 200 g of avocado, red onion, 400 g of tomatoes, chopped parsley, four tablespoons of extra virgin olive oil, lemon juice, red wine vinegar, salt and pepper to taste.

Bring the water to a boil, add the quinoa, mix, and bring back to a boil. Cook over medium heat for twelve minutes. Drain, and rinse well with cold water to stop cooking. Transfer the quinoa to a large bowl. Add all ingredients and mix well before serving.

LINGUINE ALLA MARSICANA

Ingredients for four people: 400 g of linguine, eight peeled tomatoes, 200 g of porcini mushrooms, ten sliced olives, a few tablespoons of capers, four tablespoons of extra virgin olive oil, garlic, onion, parsley, chili, salt, and pepper to taste.

Let the porcini mushrooms soak for a few hours before boiling them. Sauté the chopped garlic and onion in hot oil for a couple of minutes, then add the chopped mushrooms, chopped capers, and olives; fry for a couple of minutes. Finally, add the chopped tomato. Separately, boil the pasta in boiling salted water, drain, and season with the sauce prepared separately. Sprinkle with chopped fresh parsley and serve.

GREEN MILLET

Ingredients for four people: 400 grams of millet, 200 g of broccoli, 200 g of Romanesco cabbage, 200 g of white cauliflower, 200 g of potatoes, four tablespoons of very seasoned grated parmesan, four tablespoons of extra virgin olive oil, garlic, four tablespoons of toasted, and salted pistachios, salt, and pepper to taste.

Wash the millet in a fine mesh colander and toast it in a pan. Pour double its volume of salted water and boil it for fifteen minutes until it absorbs all the liquid. Boil the broccoli, potatoes, and cabbage in salted water, and blend them with a little of their cooking water until it forms a thick cream. Add grated parmesan, pistachios, pepper, and some oil sautéed with a few cloves of garlic.

MILLET WITH BROCCOLI AND TOMATOES

Ingredients for four people: 400 g of shelled millet, 400 g of broccoli florets, 400 g of cherry tomatoes, four tablespoons of extra virgin olive oil, garlic, salt, and pepper to taste.

Microwave the vegetables on full power for four to five minutes. Meanwhile, boil the millet in salted water for about ten to fifteen minutes. Drain and mix it with the vegetables; season with salt, pepper, and a drizzle of oil.

WOODSMAN SOUP

Ingredients for four people: 400 g of pasta, 300 g of lentils, 300 g of mushrooms, onion, cloves, bay leaves, garlic, parsley, four tablespoons of extra virgin olive oil, salt, and pepper to taste.

Boil the lentils with some bay leaves and an onion battened with a clove after soaking them for six hours in unsalted water. While the lentils are cooking, sauté the mushrooms in a sautéed garlic, with salt and pepper, after having cleaned, and slicing them. When the lentils are almost cooked, add the pasta and salt. Add the mushrooms. Sprinkle with chopped fresh parsley and serve.

PASTA SOUP

Ingredients for four people: 400 g of ditalini (a type of pasta), 500 g of a mix of vegetables (leek, potato, and peas), vegetable broth, aromatic herbs to taste (bay leaves, parsley, thyme, marjoram, etc.), salt and pepper to taste.

Wash, and slice the leek, cut the potato into cubes, and eventually defrost the peas (or soak them in water for at least six hours). Boil all the ingredients in the vegetable broth and serve on the table. Alternatively, you can start with the vegetables and add pasta or rice after ten to fifteen minutes. To give more flavor, you can add a bay leaf during cooking or other aromatic herbs to taste (parsley, marjoram, etc.).

BROCCOLI, QUINOA, TOFU, AND LIME SOUP

Ingredients for four people: 400 g of quinoa, 150 g of natural tofu, 400 g of broccoli, 400 g of leeks, four tablespoons of extra virgin olive oil, lime juice, salt, and pepper to taste.

Wash, clean, and slice the leek. Rinse the broccoli and cut the florets. Put the vegetables in a large pot and cover them with the boiling vegetable broth. Bring to a simmer, and, when it starts to boil, add the previously rinsed quinoa. Cook the soup over low heat for fifteen minutes, until the vegetables are tender, and the quinoa has swollen. While the soup is cooking, cut the tofu into pieces about 1 cm apart. Add the tofu to the soup one minute before removing it from the heat. Remove the soup from the heat and squeeze the lime juice over it. Stir, divide into serving dishes, and serve.

RICE AND POTATO SOUP

Ingredients for four people: 400 g of rice, 400 g of new potatoes, four tablespoons of extra virgin olive oil, parsley, onion, broth, salt, and pepper to taste.

In a saucepan, fry the onion with the oil. As soon as it becomes golden, add the potatoes cut into small pieces and the rice. Mix well, cover with broth, season with a little salt and pepper, and cook over moderate heat, adding more broth if necessary. When the rice is ready, add some chopped parsley, and serve to the table.

SPINACH AND RICE SOUP

Ingredients for four people: 400 g of rice, 400 g of spinach, some chopped basil leaves, garlic, 50 g of grated aged pecorino, four tablespoons of extra virgin olive oil, salt.

Boil the chopped spinach in water with the rice. Add the basil, salt, garlic, pecorino cheese, and oil. Keep on the heat for two more minutes while stirring and serve on the table.

BARLEY WITH VEGETABLES

Ingredients for four people: 400 g of pearl barley, one and a half kg of a mix of vegetables (carrots, broccoli, artichokes, chicory), four tablespoons of extra virgin olive oil, onion, vegetable broth, salt and pepper to taste.

Wash, clean, and slice the vegetables. Fry the onion in oil until wilted, and add the vegetables, stirring for a few minutes. Add the pearl barley, and mix. Add double broth to the saucepan's contents and simmer for thirty to forty minutes or until the barley is tender. Add boiling broth from time to time as needed.

PASTA ALLA MONTANARA

Ingredients for four people: 400 g of pasta, 300 g of champignons, 300 g of cabbage, 300 g of leeks, four peeled tomatoes, four tablespoons of grated swiss cheese, four tablespoons of extra virgin olive oil, garlic, salt, and pepper to taste.

Wash, clean, and slice the vegetables and mushrooms. Sauté them in hot oil with garlic for a few minutes. Add the chopped tomato, salt, and pepper. Cook for thirty minutes. Meanwhile, boil the pasta in salted water, drain it, and season it with the sauce prepared separately. Sprinkle with grated swiss cheese before serving.

SPRING RICE

Ingredients for four people: 400 g of rice, 400 g of peas, 400 g of a mix of carrots, onion, and cherry tomatoes, four tablespoons of extra virgin olive oil, salt, and pepper to taste.

Boil the rice in salted water. While cooking, place a metal colander over the pot containing the sliced vegetables and peas. Cover with a lid to steam the vegetables while the rice cooks. Drain and mix the rice with the vegetables; season with oil, salt, and pepper before serving.

PORRIDGE WITH FRUIT

Ingredients for four people: 250 g of oat flakes, 1.5 liters of water, 600 g of fruit cut into small pieces, one jar of plain yogurt or soy (optional).

Boil the water in the kettle and place the oat flakes in a bowl. When the water boils, pour it over the oat flakes, and mix. Wait three minutes for the oats to absorb the water; add the chopped fruit and a spoonful of plain yogurt. Harder fruit (such as apples and pears) can also be added to the boiling water at the beginning to soften. Alternatively, you can leave the oat flakes to soak in orange juice for a few hours without having to cook them.

LEMON AND GINGER QUINOA

Ingredients for four people: 400 g of quinoa, 400 g of chickpeas (weight after soaking), chopped parsley, lemon juice, ten olives sliced into slices, ginger powder, a few bay leaves, four tablespoons of oil extra virgin olive oil, salt.

Boil the quinoa in salted water and the chickpeas separately in water with bay leaves. Drain, then remove the bay leaves and mix before serving.

RICE WITH SOY SAUCE

Ingredients for four people: 400 g of rice, 400 g of soybeans (fresh weight or after soaking), 600 g of peeled tomatoes, four tablespoons of extra virgin olive oil, onion, salt, and pepper to taste.

Blanch the soybeans for a few minutes in salted water. Drain, and squeeze them. Brown the onion, and, when wilted, add the soybeans, and sauté for a few minutes. Add the tomatoes and cook for thirty minutes. Separately, boil the rice, drain it once cooked, and season it with the sauce prepared separately.

RICE WITH CHICKPEAS

Ingredients for four people: 400 g of rice, 300 g of dried chickpeas, bay leaves, onion, parsley, vegetable broth, four tablespoons of extra virgin olive oil, salt, and chili powder.

Soak the chickpeas twelve hours in advance, drain, and boil them for forty-five minutes in the broth, along with the chopped onion and bay leaves. After this time, adjust the broth, bring it back to a boil, and add the rice. Cover, and cook for ten to fifteen minutes. Drain and season with chopped parsley, oil, and chili powder.

BEANS AND BROCCOLI RICE

Ingredients for four people: 400 g of long grain rice, 600 g of boiled white beans, 600 g of broccoli, broth, four tablespoons of aged parmesan, fresh basil, four tablespoons of extra virgin olive oil, salt, and pepper to taste.

If you are using canned beans, rinse them in a colander under running water. Put the beans and rice in a deep saucepan or skillet; add the salt, and cover with the broth. Bring to a boil. When the liquid boils, adjust the heat to continue to boil steadily but not vigorously, and place a lid over the pot. Cook for five to seven minutes until the rice begins to turn tender but not yet thoroughly boiled. Cut the broccoli, and separate the florets, slicing the stems to the thickness you prefer. When the rice begins to become tender, add the broccoli, adjusting the broth as well if necessary. Cover the pot and cook until the rice and broccoli are tender. You can continue cooking until the rice has absorbed all the broth, checking every minute or two. Add the olive oil, parmesan, basil, and pepper.

BLACK RICE WITH PUMPKIN, CANNELLINI, AND TOFU

Ingredients for four people: 400 g of black rice, 300 g of pumpkin pulp, 200 g of boiled cannellini beans, 150 g of natural tofu, four tablespoons of extra virgin olive oil, sage, salt to taste.

Rinse the rice under running water and cook it according to the time indicated on the package. Drain it once it is ready and pour it into a bowl. In the meantime, cut the pumpkin pulp into cubes, transfer it to a baking dish, add the sage, a pinch of salt, a teaspoon of oil, and cook in the oven for twenty minutes at 180°C. Add the pumpkin to the rice along with the cannellini beans and crumbled tofu. Sprinkle with the remaining amount of oil, season with salt, and put on the table.

POLENTA WITH POTATOES

Ingredients for four people: 1 kg of potatoes, 200 g of corn flour, 1 liter of milk, broth, salt and pepper.

Boil the potatoes, mash and mix them with the milk. Pour everything into a medium-sized pot and place it on the stove. Wait for the mixture to boil, add the salt, and pour in the yellow flour. Stir, and cook the polenta for half an hour, adding boiling broth if necessary. In the last ten minutes, add the pepper.

POLENTA MARZOLINA

Ingredients for four people: 300 g of corn flour, 450 g of shelled fresh peas, six artichoke hearts, four tablespoons of extra virgin olive oil, onion, chopped parsley, broth, salt, and pepper to taste.

Brown the onion, add the sliced peas, artichoke hearts, parsley, salt, and pepper. Cook for a few minutes, stirring a couple of times. Add some broth and cook for about half an hour. Separately, bring some salted water to a boil, add the corn flour, stir constantly, and let it cook for thirty to forty minutes, stirring occasionally. When cooked mix the polenta, the peas, and the artichokes.

My best cooking tips for vegetables

Vegetables are the base of a healthy diet, and your goal is to eat them at least a couple of times a day, both cooked and raw. However, cooking vegetables is not as simple as it seems because there are mistakes that will make your vegetables lose flavor and nutrients. Therefore, it is better to know how to cook them best.

Here are my tips:

- Have both raw and cooked vegetables since some nutrients are destroyed by cooking, while in others some nutrients become more bioavailable. You can eat raw vegetables one day and cooked vegetable the day after or have them both at each meal.

- Minimize waste. Recycle your vegetables' cooking water and use the peel and green parts that you would normally discard to prepare vegetable broths or soups.

- Another quick and effortless way to cook vegetables is to boil them, and then blend them with an immersion blender to make a creamy soup. Season your creamy soup with extra virgin olive oil, some grated cheese, and serve them with boiled grains or whole meal bread croutons. A creamy vegetable soup can also go well with meat and fish dishes. Be aware that not all vegetables can be boiled; those with a high acidity level, such as peppers and tomatoes, tend to get spoiled if cooked in water and should be stewed instead.

- Cooking in a pan preserves most nutritional properties of your vegetables; try not to overdo the cooking so that they will remain crunchy. Carotenoids, lycopene, and other lypophilic antioxidants contained in some vegetables, such as cabbages, broccoli, and tomatoes, increase their bioavailability when vegetables are cooked in oil.

- Cabbages are one of the best vegetables if you want to get some vitamin C, but this vitamin is sensitive to high temperatures, therefore cooking will destroy most of it. Eat your cabbage raw, for instance as an ingredient of a salad. Cabbage is one of the vegetables that gives the best results when minimally cooked, not compromising its nutritional qualities.

- Don't throw away leftover vegetables, you can store them in the fridge and eat them the following day. You can simply reheat them or use them to create new dishes. For instance, you can toss them on toasted bread (or croutons) or mix them with some eggs and prepare an omelet. Leftover vegetables can also be reused as a condiment for rice or pasta, or used to prepare a salad, together with olives, olive oil, and anchovies.

- Steamed vegetables retain their nutritional properties more than boiled ones. Steaming can take longer in some cases, but it will keep the flavor of your vegetables intact.

- Vegetables that have a hard consistency will soften if you soak them into a marinade based of oil, vinegar, salt, lemon, and spices. Two hours of soaking are enough to soften them.

- In theory, you can fry any kind of vegetable. You don't necessarily need to dip them in batter or bread them before frying. Everyone knows french fries, but you can also fry cauliflower, onions, courgettes, and even stuffed zucchini flowers. But beware that this is not the healthiest cooking technique.

- Finally, did you know that you can make chips with vegetables other than potatoes? Try slicing a raw beet with a peeler. Place it on a baking sheet and put it in the oven on the highest temperature until the chips are crisp. Sprinkle a little salt, and you will discover a new and delicious dish.

Recipes with vegetables

ARTICHOKES WITH OLIVES

Ingredients for four people: 400 g of artichoke hearts, 160 g of black olives, eight tablespoons of extra virgin olive oil, lemon juice, parsley, garlic, salt and pepper to taste.

Cut the artichoke hearts in half and remove any beard. Slice them thinly and dip them in water acidulated with lemon juice. Sauté the garlic and, after a couple of minutes, add the artichokes and olives. Cook for about half an hour, possibly adding a few spoons of hot water. Just before turning off the heat, sprinkle with chopped fresh parsley and put it on the table.

CAULIFLOWER AND SPICY BROCCOLI

Ingredients for four people: 800 g of cauliflower, 800 g of broccoli, four tablespoons of extra virgin olive oil, one teaspoon of chili powder, four tablespoons of extra virgin olive oil, salt and pepper to taste.

Steam the vegetables briefly, pour them into a pan with hot oil. Add salt and pepper, cook for five to ten minutes and sprinkle with chili powder before serving.

ORANGE BRUSSELS SPROUTS

Ingredients for four people: 800 g of Brussels sprouts, 100 ml of vegetable cream, 50 g of potato starch, six to eight blond oranges, ground cloves, salt and pepper to taste.

Clean the sprouts and boil them in salted water. Drain them and let them drain well, and then brown them in hot oil. Turn them on all sides, then sprinkle them with the starch, salt, pepper, cloves powder (a little), and grated orange peel. Wet them with the orange juice and immediately add the cream. Mix everything until the bottom becomes creamy. Distribute onto plates and decorate with orange slices.

PUMPKIN CREAMY SOUP WITH CHILI PEPPER

Ingredients for four people: 1.5 kg of pumpkin, one teaspoon of chopped hot pepper, two or three handfuls of sprouts of your favorite type, thyme, salt and pepper to taste.

Cut the pumpkin pulp into chunks and boil them until it becomes soft. Blend them with enough cooking water to obtain a soft cream. Add thyme, salt, and pepper and mix. Sprinkle with the sprouts and serve.

FENNEL WITH CURRY AND LEMON

Ingredients for four people: 1 kg of fennel, 800 g of tomato sauce, curry, grated organic lemon zest, four tablespoons of extra virgin olive oil, salt and pepper to taste.

Clean the fennel, cut them into even slices, and put them in a saucepan with hot oil. Brown them on both sides and add the tomato sauce, a hint of curry, salt, and pepper. Cook for ten to fifteen minutes, stirring occasionally, and serve garnished with grated lemon zest and pepper.

SAUTÉD MUSHROOMS

Ingredients for four people: 800 g of champignon mushrooms, garlic, parsley, four tablespoons of extra virgin olive oil, salt and pepper to taste.

Wash the mushrooms well and cut them into thin slices. In a pan, sauté the garlic in the oil, add the mushrooms and cook for fifteen minutes. When cooked, add salt and pepper, then sprinkle with chopped fresh parsley before serving.

GUACAMOLE

Ingredients for four people: four small tomatoes, 200 g of avocado, four cloves of garlic, onion, four tablespoons of lime juice, two tablespoons of extra virgin olive oil, chili powder, salt and pepper to taste.

Cut the avocado in half and extract the indicated amount of pulp. The remainder can be cut into cubes and frozen. Place the pulp in a bowl and mash it until you get a creamy pulp. Wash and finely chop the garlic and onion and mix them with the avocado cream and chili powder, lime juice, oil, salt, and pepper. Mix well. Slice the tomato into cubes and add it to the cream. Stir and refrigerate at least an hour before serving.

SALAD OF BROCCOLI, STRAWBERRIES, AND BLUEBERRIES

Recipe for four people: Mix 200 g of mixed leaf salads, 200 g of raw broccoli florets, 200 g of strawberries cut into four parts, four tablespoons of blueberries, four tablespoons of chopped hazelnuts.

BAKED AUBERGINES

Ingredients for four people: 800 g of aubergine, 400 g of stale breadcrumbs, 80 g of olives, 120 g of walnut kernels, a few handfuls of capers, parsley, oregano, salt and pepper to taste.

Peel the aubergines and slice them lengthwise. Place them in a dish with salt and let them sit for half an hour. Meanwhile, mix the stale breadcrumbs with the sliced olives, parsley, oregano, capers, and chopped walnuts in a bowl. Dry the aubergines from the water they have produced in the meantime, using a clean cloth or absorbent paper. Spread the bread mixture prepared separately on each slice. Drizzle with oil, add salt and pepper and then bake at 200°C for about half an hour, with the pan covered with aluminum foil. After this time, remove the foil and continue cooking for another ten minutes. Remove from the oven and put on the table.

SWEET POTATOES WITH ROSEMARY

Ingredients for four people: 1 kg and a half of spinach, 1 kg of sweet potatoes, chopped rosemary, four tablespoons of extra virgin olive oil, salt and pepper to taste.

Peel the potatoes and cut them into cubes after washing them. Cook them in a pan with hot oil for fifteen minutes, seasoning with salt. Add the spinach and rosemary and sauté for a few minutes until the spinach wilt. Sprinkle with pepper and serve.

PEPERONATA WITH OLIVES

Ingredients for four people: 800 g of peppers, 800 g of ripe tomatoes (or peeled), 100 g of olives, six tablespoons of extra virgin olive oil, 2 tablespoons of vinegar, onion, salt and pepper.

Wash and slice the peppers and tomatoes. Sauté the onion in the hot oil until it wilts. Add the tomatoes, peppers, and olives, as well as the vinegar. Add salt and pepper and continue cooking for about half an hour before serving.

TOMATOES STUFFED WITH AVOCADO

Ingredients for four people: 800 g of Roma or San Marzano tomatoes, four avocados, four tablespoons of extra virgin olive oil, onion, chopped fresh parsley, salt.

Cut the tomatoes in half lengthwise and drain them on absorbent paper. Mash the avocado with a fork and mix it with the finely chopped onion, oil, and salt. Stuff the tomatoes with this mixture and serve with a sprinkle of parsley.

VELVET SAUCE, CAULIFLOWER, AND LENTILS

Ingredients for four people: 400 g of cabbage, 400 g of cauliflower, 160 g of dried lentils, four pieces of kombu seaweed (optional), garlic, sage, four tablespoons of extra virgin olive oil, 150 ml of sugar-free oat milk added, chopped parsley, boiling vegetable broth, salt, and pepper to taste.

Soak the lentils in plenty of cold water overnight. Cook them for thirty minutes in a liter of water with the kombu seaweed and garlic. Once cooked, cover them and let them cool. Season with a little oil, salt, and pepper, and keep them aside. Wash the cabbage and cut it into thin strips. Clean the cauliflower and divide it into small florets.

Cut the sage leaves into small pieces. In a saucepan, heat two tablespoons of oil with the sage, add the cauliflower and the cabbage. Add the salt, mix, add the broth, and cook with the cover on for ten minutes. Remove the lid and finish cooking for another five minutes. Reduce to cream with the hand blender. Put it back on the heat, add the oat drink, cook for a few more minutes. Season with salt and pepper. Serve the soup hot in individual bowls, arrange the lentils in the center and sprinkle with the chopped parsley and a drizzle of oil.

PUMPKIN GRATIN WITH TOASTED DRIED FRUIT

Ingredients for four people: 800 g of pumpkin, fresh sage, four tablespoons of extra virgin olive oil, 80 ml of vegetable cream, 40 g of hazelnuts, 40 g of pecans or pistachios, four tablespoons of very seasoned parmesan, salt and pepper to taste.

Heat the oven to 230°C. Chop the squash in a blender or use a grater. Chop a few sage leaves. Put the pumpkin in a baking dish. Add the sage, a tablespoon of olive oil, and a sprinkle of salt and pepper. Pour the cream over the mixture. Cover the pan with aluminum foil and cook for fifteen to twenty minutes, until the squash is tender and the cream thicker. Chop the walnuts and grate the parmesan. When the pumpkin is tender, uncover the pan, sprinkle with the grated parmesan cheese and the dried fruit. Return to the oven and cook uncovered until the top is lightly browned, about five minutes longer. Let it cool for a minute or two before serving.

ONION SOUP

Ingredients for four people: 600 g of blond onions, four tablespoons of white flour, four tablespoons of grated parmesan, 400 g of sliced homemade bread, four tablespoons of extra virgin olive oil, broth, salt and pepper to taste.

Boil some water to make the broth. Meanwhile, slice the onions very thin and sauté them in oil over low heat. When they become brown, add the flour, making it fall from a colander not to form lumps and stirring constantly. Add the broth to the onions, one ladle at a time. Season with salt and cook for half an hour. Meanwhile, toast the slices of homemade bread and place them in a crock cup. Sprinkle with the grated cheese and cover them with the onions prepared separately. Place in a preheated oven at 200°C for five minutes or until the soup is browned.

My best tips for cooking fish

F ish is not only a pillar of the Italian cuisine and of the Mediterranean diet, but it is also a fundamental food for staying healthy. It is rich in protein, minerals (such as phosphorus), vitamins, and especially polyunsaturated fats such as omega 3 which is useful for keeping blood cholesterol and triglyceride levels at bay preventing cardiovascular disease. For these reasons, my personal recommendation is to eat fish at least a couple of times a week. The best fish is the high-fat one, typically bluefish.

There are many ways to cook fish, here below you will find the most common preparation techniques that work well for this type of food.

Raw. This is a type of preparation used mainly for appetizers, such as carpaccio. For the latter, use very fresh fish, preserved in compliance with all hygiene rules. Sushi is a perfect example of raw fish that manages to become an exciting dish. You can also prepare salmon or tuna mousse by blending it and serving it with puff pastry or other ingredients.

Poached or braised. This cooking technique is perfect for cooking hake, snapper, cod, and sea bream. The goal of this cooking technique is to keep the fish hydrated so that it will not lose its flavor. It is vital that you never boil your fish, but to cook it at a low temperature and generously season the fish after removing the skin.

With grains. Fish works well with pasta, rice, couscous and other grains. You can use it to prepare a pasta sauce, like "spaghetti alle vongole" or "penne al salmone" or a seafood risotto. You can also prepare ravioli stuffed with fish mixed with herbs.

In the pan or roasted. Cooking in a pan, possibly together

with some vegetables, is perfect for thin fish and fish fillets, such as the classic plaice fillet you can find in all supermarkets. Pan cooking is suitable for most kinds of fish, as is grilling. However, large fish slices and fillets (especially those from large fish such as swordfish) may give better results when roasted. You can roast your fish in a hot oven from start to finish or sear your fish on one side in a baking dish, finishing cooking it in the oven or under the grill. Fish roasting is a pretty fast technique which usually takes fifteen to twenty minutes.

Baked. Baking a fish in foil means baking the fish in the oven

after wrapping it around a material to trap both water and the flavors. The latter is usually aluminum foil, but it is better if you opt for parchment paper, as aluminum is toxic. Cook your fish together with some salt and pepper and lots of ground herbs. When the fish is ready, just look at the foil. When it stops swelling, the fish will be cooked to perfection.

Crust baking. The principle behind cooking in a crust is the

same for foil, but instead of wrapping up your food in aluminum foil or parchment paper, you wrap your fish in bread, puff pastry, or even salt. This cooking technique is suitable for fish such as the sea bass or the sea bream. Remember to leave the skin, especially if you cook you fish in a salt crust, to prevent the fish from becoming excessively salty.

Frying. This is one of the most common and easiest techniques to cook fish, although you should eat fried fish only once in a while since it is not ideal for your diet and health. Fry your fish in plenty of hot oil after patting it with flour or breadcrumbs for a few minutes. When the fish is ready, let the excess oil drain on an absorbent cloth. You can fry all kinds of fish and seafood.

Steamed. You can steam your fish in a steamer by putting it into a colander that you will place on top of a pot with boiling water. I recommend that you also steam some chopped vegetables together with your fish. Vegetables that contain a lot of water, such as green leafy vegetables, zucchini, and fresh tomatoes, will release liquids and contribute to the formation of steam. You can also mix them with other starchy vegetables, such as potatoes, but you will probably need to add some liquid later during cooking.

Steaming fish takes about the same time it takes to soften the vegetables. If you want the vegetables just to be slightly tender, toss them until they are still somewhat crunchy to eat. Add enough water to keep them from sticking.

If the vegetable juices are boiling in the pan's bottom, do not add any more liquid. Otherwise, wet slightly. If you want something more like a stew, add enough liquid to give the vegetables a "gravy-like" texture.

Large fish fillets, shrimp, clams, and mussels are ideal for steaming - they cook quickly and stay moist. Arrange them on top of the vegetables, sprinkle them with salt and pepper, and cover the pan with a lid. Steam until the fish is cooked, checking it from time to time, adding more liquid if necessary. When the fish is ready, the vegetables will be, too. Serve on a plate with the fish, and sprinkle with the juices left in the pan.

Recipes with fish

MACKEREL WITH OLIVES

Ingredients for four people: 800 g of filleted mackerel, 80 g of sliced olives, onion, 800 g of ripe tomatoes, oregano, bay leaves, parsley, 50 g of extra virgin olive oil, salt and pepper to taste.

Brown the onion in hot oil, add the olives and tomatoes. Let it cook for about thirty minutes, stirring occasionally. Meanwhile, turn on the oven to 200°C, bake the fish together with the sauce prepared separately, a sprinkling of oregano, and chopped bay leaves. Cook for about half an hour in a pan covered with aluminum foil, serve hot on the table.

PRAWN SKEWERS

Ingredients for four people: 1.5 kg of prawns, 400 g of avocado, 500 g of artichoke hearts, 100 ml of lemon juice, 50 g of extra virgin olive oil, one teaspoon of Worcestershire sauce, tabasco, oregano, garlic, salt and pepper to taste.

Prepare the marinade by blending the following ingredients in the blender: oil, Worcestershire sauce, tabasco, oregano, finely chopped garlic, salt, and pepper. Cut the avocado into large pieces, and the artichoke hearts in half. Place them in the freshly prepared sauce along with the shrimp and leave to marinate for about 2 hours. Put the shrimp, artichokes, and avocado on one or more skewers, and roast them in the oven for six to seven minutes at 180°C, after sprinkling the marinade on top of them.

SWORDFISH AL SALMORIGLIO

Ingredients for four people: 800 g of swordfish, 50 g of extra virgin olive oil, lemon juice, oregano, and fresh parsley, salt and pepper to taste.

Mix the lemon juice with olive oil, salt, and pepper. Add the chopped oregano and parsley. Grill the fish two to three minutes on each side, and then season it with the sauce prepared on the side before serving.

SCAMPI AL CARTOCCIO

Ingredients for four people: 600 g of scampi, four eggs, flour, four tablespoons of extra virgin olive oil, parsley, five to six lemon wedges, salt and pepper to taste.

Beat the eggs in a bowl with the salt. Dip the scampi in the egg and then in the flour. Wrap in parchment paper, wet with oil, and bake in the oven at 180°C for about twenty to thirty minutes. Serve with a few lemon wedges.

CUTTLEFISH WITH SPINACH

Ingredients for four people: 600 g of frozen cuttlefish (thawed weight), 800 g of fresh spinach, garlic, onion, 50 g of extra virgin olive oil, brandy, salt and pepper to taste.

Thaw the cuttlefish and, in the meantime, sauté the garlic and onion in the oil. At this point, you can add the cuttlefish, salt, pepper, and let it brown. Add a little brandy, and let it evaporate. Cover, and cook for thirty-five minutes, adding a little water from time to time if the sauce gets dry. After this time, add the spinach leaves, and sauté together with the cuttlefish. Cook for another fifteen minutes before serving.

My best tips for cooking eggsEggs are an alternative to meat and contains important protein. The egg is an embryonic cell and, as such, has exceptional nutritional power, and contains high-quality protein. It is also an easy-to-digest food, very versatile when it comes to cooking it, and it can be used in numerous preparations, from appetizers to desserts. Although eggs have often been accused of being unhealthy due to their high cholesterol content, it now seems that the polyunsaturated fats they contain can offset this disadvantage. Furthermore, the human body is perfectly able to regulate cholesterol production based on the amount consumed in the diet.The egg white is rich in protein and low in fat, while the yolk contains unsaturated fat. Rich in vitamins and minerals, eggs represent a complete food with a medium energy content that provides all the amino acids the body needs. They are a choline source, an amino acid that is protective for neuronal and cardiovascular health, which is a component of phosphatidylcholine, an essential constituent of cell membranes. A metabolite of choline, betaine, reduces the accumulation of homocysteine, a cardiovascular risk factor. The yolk contains carotenoids (but only if the poultry were fed with corn). The fact that the egg also contains fats makes carotenoids even more bioavailable since they are fat-soluble compounds.

Not just omelets: egg preparation guide

When buying eggs, check how fresh they are. You just need to dip an egg in saltwater and if it sinks, it is fresh. If the egg is not fresh, it will instead surface a few millimeters or float.

There are various ways to cook eggs: hard-boiled, scrambled, soft-boiled, etc. It is also possible to cook them in boiling water, without the shell. To prevent the egg white from flaking, add a couple of tablespoons of vinegar to the cooking water. In Italy we call this technique in a funny way: "uova affogate," which literally means "drowned egg." Soft -boiled cooking ('egg á la coque') involves boiling the egg for three to four minutes maximum. Place the egg in an egg cup with the pointed side facing up and eat it with a teaspoon after removing the top of the shell and sprinkling with a pinch of salt. Scrambled or fried eggs represent another possibility. Choose oils that resist heat, such as peanut or extra virgin olive oil. Another way to use eggs is to prepare a baked omelet.

Never store eggs with a dirty shell because the latter is very porous and will let the impurities pass through it. You can also boil cracked eggs if you rub their surface with some lemon juice in advance.

Recipes with eggs

BAKED EGGS WITH AVOCADO

Ingredients for four people: four avocados, eight eggs, chili, salt and pepper, fresh basil.

Set the oven to 225°C. Cut the avocados in half. Remove the avocados from their peel and place the halves in a baking dish. Break an egg on top of each half. At this point, you can season with salt, pepper, chili, and chopped basil. Bake in the oven for about fifteen minutes.

EGGS WITH VINEGAR

Ingredients for four people: eight eggs, eight anchovy fillets in oil, four tablespoons of extra virgin olive oil, vinegar.

Grease a baking dish with oil, break the eggs into it, and cook them in the oven at 180°C until the egg white has congealed. Serve the eggs sprinkled with the chopped anchovies and soaked for a few minutes in the vinegar.

MUSTARD EGGS

Ingredients for four people: eight eggs, four tablespoons of grated parmesan, four tablespoons of cooking cream, a little mustard, four tablespoons of extra virgin olive oil, salt and pepper to taste.

Grease a baking dish with oil, sprinkle it with grated parmesan cheese, and break the eggs on top. Separately, mix the mustard, cream, salt, and pepper. Pour everything over the eggs and bake at 180°C for fifteen minutes.

EGGS WITH GYPSY

Ingredients for four people: eight eggs, 400 g of peppers of various colors, garlic, oregano, four tablespoons of extra virgin olive oil, salt and pepper to taste.

Wash and dry the peppers, toast them on the plate, turn them on all sides until their surface is darker and crumpled (but not burned). Peel them and remove both the seeds and the white stalks they have inside. Cut them into thin strips, sauté them in a pan with oil and minced garlic. Turn them in the sauté pan over low heat, sprinkling them with oregano. Finally, place them in a baking dish. Place two shelled eggs in the center of the pan, season with salt and pepper, and bake at 180°C until the yolks begin to veil.

SCRAMBLED EGGS WITH MUSHROOMS AND BREAD

Ingredients for four people: eight eggs, four slices of homemade bread, champignon mushrooms, vegetable broth, four tablespoons of extra virgin olive oil, two tablespoons of vegetable cream, garlic, salt, pepper, four tablespoons of aged parmesan and chives.

Toast the bread, clean and slice the mushrooms. Bring the broth to a boil. Put a tablespoon of oil in a pan together with a clove of garlic, peeled and crushed. Let it brown, and then remove it from the pan. Add the mushrooms, a pinch of salt, two tablespoons of broth, and cook for ten minutes over medium heat. Add more broth if the cooking juices become too dry. When cooked, add the cream and the pepper. Mix then turn off the heat and keep covered. Pour a little oil into a pan. Break the eggs into the pan and mix with a wooden spoon. Add half the parmesan, and finish cooking. Put a portion of eggs on the bread, add the mushrooms, sprinkle with parmesan, chopped chives, and serve.

How to prepare sugar-free desserts

Cooking sweets without sugar seems like a contradiction: sweets are meant to contain sugar! Not exactly. In nature, there are many sweet substances, for example, in fruit. You can then use the latter, or concentrated apple juice, to sweeten a dessert without resorting to sugar. By doing so, you will also add vitamins and minerals to your dessert.

I would also like to underline that we are now used to perceiving a food rich in sweeteners as "sweet." In reality, the palate can be "trained" so that you can gradually appreciate even less intense sweet flavors. Therefore, I do not recommend using some types of artificial sweeteners, such as aspartame or saccharin, because they give 1,000 to 10,000 times more flavor than regular cooking sugar.

Many recipes I've found in blogs or cookbooks contain coconut sugar. I don't think it's a good idea to use it; While everyone claims that it has a lower glycemic index than sucrose (the regular cooking sugar), coconut sugar is still 80% sucrose. You can read more about this in my blog[2].

I also advise against honey, unless you use very little of it, and make sure you buy it from a known manufacturer. Honey is one of the most adulterated foods there is; the cheaper ones are in fact, concentrated fructose syrup. A common scam, in short, since it is complicated to

---

[2] Coconut sugar: you can't have your cake, and eat it, too! https://www.gianlucatognon.com/coconut-palm-sugar-cant-cake-eat/

distinguish real honey from fructose syrup.[3] The latter also does not contain vitamins or minerals like natural honey. Agave syrup is also concentrated fructose.[4] That's why it's so sweet! Fructose is potentially sweeter than sugar, and you can theoretically use less of it. The metabolism of fructose is unregulated as well as glucose, so this sugar contributes more to the fat mass formation.

To use stevia is instead, a better idea since it is not sweeter than common sucrose, it has no calories, and you can use it for baking. However, you will not need any sugar or other sweetener to prepare most of the recipes that follow.

---

[3] Would you lying to me, honey? Honey is not as healthy as you think. https://www.gianlucatognon.com/would-you-lie-to-me-honey/

[4] Agave syrup: when the dress does not make the monk. https://www.gianlucatognon.com/agave-syrup-wolf-sheeps-clothes/

Sugar-free dessert recipes

AVOCADO AND PEAR CREAM

Ingredients for four people: 200 g of avocado pulp, 300 g of pear pulp, two tablespoons of lemon juice, two oranges, two tablespoons of grated dark chocolate.

Cut the pear and avocado pulp (both just removed from the fridge) into chunks, blend them with the freshly squeezed lemon, and orange juice until smooth. Spread the mix in a bowl, and then decorate with grated chocolate. Serve immediately.

BANANA BISCUITS WITHOUT SUGAR

Ingredients: two to three ripe bananas, two cups of oat flakes, one cup of chopped dates, 1/3 cup of extra virgin olive oil, one teaspoon of vanilla flavoring.

Turn on the oven, and let it heat up to 200°C. Meanwhile, mash the bananas, and mix them with the other ingredients in a bowl. Let it sit for a quarter of an hour, and then spread it all out on a baking sheet lined with parchment paper with the help of a spoon: a biscuit for each spoonful. Bake for twenty minutes or until the cookies are golden brown.

FLOUR-FREE BISCUITS

Ingredients: 50 g of oat flakes, 50 g of puffed rice, one ripe banana, two tablespoons of raisins, one tablespoon of chocolate chips, two tablespoons of chopped almonds, two tablespoons of chopped hazelnuts.

Mash the banana with a fork until creamy. Add the other ingredients and mix well. Line a baking sheet with parchment paper, and distribute piles of the prepared mixture on it, trying to give them a round cookie shape. Bake in the oven at 180°C for twenty minutes.

PASTRY WITHOUT SUGAR

Ingredients for a single layer: 300 grams of semi-whole meal flour, 130 grams of butter, grated lemon zest, three tablespoons of concentrated apple juice, two eggs.

Mix the flour with the previously softened butter. Add the other ingredients and continue to knead until it is entirely amalgamated and form a dough. Wrap the latter in cling wrap, and let it sit in the refrigerator for at least half an hour before using it as a base for your desserts.

SUGAR-FREE APPLE CAKE

Ingredients: three tablespoons of corn starch, one tablespoon of chopped cinnamon (optional), 350 ml of unsweetened apple juice, six grated apples, two layers of sugar-free short crust pastry (see the previous recipe).

Preheat the oven to 200°C. Mix the cornstarch with the cinnamon and a quarter of the apple juice. In a saucepan over medium heat, mix the grated apples with the rest of the apple juice until smooth. Combine with the other ingredients and add more cornstarch to increase the consistency of the dough. Put the short crust pastry in a pan, add the apple mixture, and cover with a second layer of short crust pastry. Bake in the oven for about forty-five minutes.

NUTS WITH HAZELNUT BUTTER

Ingredients: half a cup of unsalted peanut butter, three tablespoons of powdered milk, three tablespoons of coconut flakes (or grated coconut), five tablespoons of oat flakes, two to three tablespoons of apple juice without sugar.

Mix and work all the ingredients by hand until you form a compact dough. Form a series of balls of the size you want and place them in the refrigerator for a few hours before consuming them. Store in the fridge.

OAT NUGGETS

Ingredients: three tablespoons of oat flakes, three tablespoons of unsweetened cocoa powder, two tablespoons of date concentrate (or crumbled dried dates), three tablespoons of peanut cream, four tablespoons of grated coconut (or coconut flakes).

Mix all the ingredients carefully, except the coconut. Shape into balls and roll them in coconut. Store in the refrigerator.

SUGAR-FREE CAKE

Ingredients: two cups of raisins, three cups of water, two eggs, three tablespoons of sweetener (for example, stevia), one sachet of baking powder, one tablespoon of vanilla extract, half a teaspoon of salt, half a teaspoon of nutmeg, two cups of semi-whole meal white flour, one cup of chopped walnuts, ¾ of a cup of extra virgin olive oil, one cup of unsweetened apple juice.

Heat the oven to 200°C. Mix the raisins with the water in a small pan and cook until they absorb the whole water. Let it cool down. Put the other ingredients (except the walnuts) in a bowl and mix until you get a smooth dough. Add the walnuts and raisins, and place on a baking sheet lined with parchment paper. Bake for about an hour.

COCONUT ICE CREAM

Ingredients: two cups of coconut milk with no added sugar, ¼ cup of coconut oil, two tablespoons of passion fruit extract (or other exotic fruit), one tablespoon of lime juice, one tablespoon of flakes or coconut extract.

Mix all the ingredients and blend. Chill in the refrigerator for at least an hour. Put everything back in the ice cream maker and follow the instructions in the appliance manual. Keep in the freezer, and then leave it out for five to ten minutes before consuming.

PEACH SORBET

Ingredients: three ripe peaches, ice cubes.

Peel the peaches and cut them into chunks. Place them in a food container suitable for the freezer. Leave them in the freezer for at least one night and then put them in a blender with some ice cubes. Blend until you get a soft cream. Check the instructions of your blender to make sure it is suitable for blending ice. Stir well and serve.

How to use herbs and spices to flavor your dishes

erbs are a typical ingredient of the Mediterranean cuisine. Among the best known, I would like to mention sage, rosemary, oregano, and thyme are all typical plants of the Mediterranean basin. In Italian cuisine, basil, parsley, rosemary, thyme, oregano, and sage are also widely used such as hot pepper. Basil, for example, is used for the preparation of the very famous pesto. Other cuisines, such as the Moroccan one, favor using spices, such as saffron, cinnamon, ginger, turmeric, pepper, and paprika. Among the most used, we find paprika, very common in North African countries, and then introduced in Spain by the Moors.

Pepper is also ubiquitous in Italian and Spanish cuisines. The Arabs instead introduced the use of saffron in Spain. Finally, in Greek cuisine, fennel and sesame seeds are also used a lot.

These aromas contain a large number of health-promoting phytochemicals, such as capsanthin, a carotenoid found in paprika. Other antioxidants are released when herbs are cut or chopped. Herbs and spices allow you to add more flavor to foods, reducing table salt and glutamate.

Some herbs hold up well when cooked while retaining a strong flavor, such as oregano, rosemary, marjoram, sage, thyme, tarragon, wild fennel, and chives. Laurel also belongs to this category, indispensable in the composition of the aromatic bunch to prepare the broth. Given its intense aroma, many people remove bay leaves after cooking. Other, more delicate herbs spoil more easily during cooking. These include basil, parsley, Pimpinella, sorrel, chervil, and mint, which you should add after cooking. Our gastronomic culture has favored some varieties, giving rise to combinations that have become classics, such as roast with rosemary, sardines, and fennel, and basil with tomato.

Bay leaves and dill go perfectly with many seafood dishes. Chervil is perfect for adding more flavor to white meat, eggs, and salads. Coriander complements stews, fish, and sauces. Parsley gives flavor to everything: soups, sauces, vegetables, meat, fish, and is essential for preparing a green sauce. Rosemary also goes perfectly with baked potatoes and fish. Sage is ideal with chicken, and rabbit, as well as with rice, gnocchi, and ravioli. Legumes also go well with sage, as you will discover if you taste beans all'uccelletto during a trip to Tuscany. Mint is used in sauces, with lamb, in salads, desserts, and herbal teas. Basil, an essential ingredient for pesto, enriches dressings, salads, sauces, pizza, oil, and vinegar with flavor. Oregano adds flavor to raw tomatoes, grilled meat, fish, and even bread. Its flavor intensifies once dried. Marjoram, used in Ligurian cuisine, is pleasant in soups, fillings, and roasts. Thyme aromatizes all slow-cooking dishes, sauces, vegetables, and roasts; it is also used to perfume cheeses and prepare liqueurs. Why don't you start enriching your kitchen with some aromatic herbs you didn't know or have never used before? You will be amazed by your renewed culinary skills!

How to use vegetable oils

While shopping, you will often come across an astounding array of oils that crowd the supermarket shelves. Unfortunately, a great deal of myths and misinformation have spread on the internet about the correct use of edible oils. Therefore, it is legitimate to wonder which are the best oils to buy and how to use them correctly. This guide will help you learn about the origin, use, and benefits of different oil types.

Oils such as rapeseed, corn, cottonseed, olive, safflower, soybean, and sunflower oils come from the respective plants' seeds. Additionally, some foods are naturally high in oils, such as nuts, olives, avocados, and some fish (e.g., cod liver).

Two examples of relatively new oils on the market are avocado oil and coconut oil. Avocado oil is rich in monounsaturated fats, the same as olive oil, and has a high smoke point, making it potentially suitable for cooking. Although you can use coconut oil for cooking at high temperatures, its high saturated fat content suggests moderation. A recent analysis of the scientific literature on coconut oil's health effects indicated that coconut oil might raise "bad" cholesterol levels. However, this doesn't seem to be true for virgin coconut oil.

- Extra virgin olive oil combines taste with the health properties of monounsaturated fats. It has a low to moderate smoke point, and its flavor is lost with cooking. Therefore, it is best to use it for raw or slightly heated dishes, including sautéing, if not prolonged for a long time.

- Soybean, sunflower, corn oils work only for seasoning, but consider they don't have the same health properties as olive oil.
- Walnut, linseed, and sesame oils are used raw, mainly as a flavoring, and have some health properties.

Other oils are also suitable for cooking, for example:

- Rapeseed oil has a neutral flavor. Its high smoke point makes this oil a suitable choice for cooking and frying. Most canola oils on the market are highly refined, which means they don't have as many antioxidants like olive oil.
- Peanut oil has a high smoke point, which makes it resistant to cooking over high heat.
- Grapeseed oil is also suitable for cooking at high temperatures

Refined oils have a greater smoke point than unrefined oils. In case you did not know, the smoke point is the temperature at which they start to produce smoke when heated, and it is an indication of the temperature at which you can cook them without spoiling them. Although refined oils' heat resistance is higher, you should avoid them because the refining process involves harmful chemical processes.

The nutritional value of extra virgin olive oil

Unlike other oil species in which the most abundant fat is linoleic acid (unsaturated), oleic acid (monounsaturated) prevails in olive oil, considered the most effective fatty acid in reducing blood cholesterol levels and cardiovascular disease. Oleic acid is one of the most digestible fatty acids, both for its organoleptic characteristics and because it stimulates conditioned reflexes within the gastrointestinal tract that favor pancreatic secretion. Oleic acid easily passes through the intestinal mucosa and is rapidly absorbed. It can also stimulate bile secretion, which is essential for the absorption of fats in the intestine.

The best effects on health belong above all to extra-virgin and virgin olive oil. Since it contains more oleic acid than polyunsaturated fats, olive oil is more resistant to high-temperature cooking. However, the heat considerably reduces the beneficial properties of the oil, which loses many vitamins and bioactive compounds at high temperatures. However, it is worth mentioning another fatty acid which may be responsible for the beneficial properties of olive oil: squalene. This fatty acid is more concentrated in olive oil than other oils (see the table below) and appears to play a role in preventing cardiovascular disease, diabetes, and cancer.

Type of oil	Squalene content (mg / 100 g)
Olive	136-708
Corn	19-36
Peanut	13-49
Soy	7-17
Sunflower	8-19
Rapeseed	28

Olive oil is rich in many natural substances: chlorophyll, carotenoids, tocopherols, polyphenols, and others. The presence of bioactive compounds, including vitamin E, makes olive oil a stable product, at least in terms of conservation for much longer times than its shelf life (generally indicated in a calendar year), as these compounds protect it from rancidity. The presence of polyphenols allows a further inhibition of the oxidative processes responsible for premature cellular aging. Furthermore, polyphenols contribute to the improvement of the organoleptic characteristics of the oil.

Congratulations!

I want to thank you for completing this journey of discovering how you can improve your diet and make permanent changes to your lifestyle. I hope you have found this book interesting and that above all, it has provided you with exciting ideas for changing your approach to nutrition, weight loss, and to be able to maintain it over time.

I hope my book has increased your awareness that diets are not effective for losing weight and that it is much better to become aware of what and why you eat. Being aware of how much sugar in what we ingest every day contains is also essential. I sincerely hope I have given you all the information you need to make yourself independent in managing your diet.

In this book, I discussed several ways to help manage hunger. I hope I have given you all the tools you need to distinguish real hunger (i.e., when your body asks you to eat something because it needs it), from nervous hunger, when you eat only out of boredom, stress, gluttony, or because the people around you are eating. I've done my best to give you many tips on what to do to combat emotional hunger. I'd also like to know which one is the most effective or if you've discovered any new ones.

If you like my recipes, I'm sure you will enjoy cooking and posting pictures of your delicacies on social media. The secret to doing something super is to have fun while doing it. Cooking and socializing is fun. You can cook with your whole family and strengthen your bond. Maybe either you or a member of your family will turn this passion into a job in the future.

I thought I'd write this book for people who have little time for continuous physical activity or going to the gym. However, I hope that you can take the time to move more. Always search the web or the App Store for new fitness apps that you can use at home (even with just two cases of water), and don't hesitate to contact me for updates and suggestions. It doesn't take much to change your habits, and if I've managed to integrate even one more positive habit into your daily routine, then I'll have achieved my goal.

I am always available to help you. It is the least I can do to thank you for reading this book. You can contact me using the contact form on my website[5] or use my fan page on Facebook.[6] I don't typically accept friend requests from people I don't know on my private Facebook profile. But you can send me a contact request on LinkedIn, and I will be happy to accept.[7] Finally, I hope my words have given you greater awareness of the role that food plays in your health. I am happy to have helped you and don't forget to share this new knowledge with your family and friends, because eating healthier is possible!

---

[5] My contact page: https://www.gianlucatognon.com/contact/

[6] My Facebook page: https://www.facebook.com/gianluca.tognon.4/

[7] My LinkedIn profile: https://www.linkedin.com/in/gianlucatognon/

Thank you!

I would like to thank those who have always supported me and enjoyed my blog and books. These people are my family, friends, followers, and all my clients. Without you guys, I would not have been able to go on for so many years in this profession that I never get tired of. I published this book in complete autonomy, without the contribution of a publisher or sponsor. Thanks to your support, I can continue to provide you with updated scientific information, to the best of my knowledge, and without any conflict of interest. In a world such as where we live, I believe this is important. Thank you for your contribution!

Thanks to those who will send me feedback and suggestions to improve this book.

Recommended readings

Susan Albers, 50 Ways to Soothe Yourself Without Food. New Harbinger Publications.

Susan Albers, 50 More Ways to Soothe Yourself Without Food. New Harbinger Publications.

Michael Mosley, The Fast 800: How to Combine Rapid Weight Loss and Intermittent Fasting for Long-term Health. Short Books Ed.Barry Sears, The Resolution Zone. Regan Arts Ed.